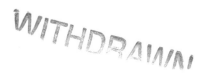

Clinical Problems in
Pediatric Urology

Clinical Problems in
Pediatric
Urology

EDITED BY

Prasad Godbole, FRCS, FRCS (Paed)

Consultant Paediatric Urologist
Sheffield Children's NHS Trust
Sheffield, UK

John P. Gearhart, MD, FACS, FAAP

Division of Paediatric Urology
Professor & Chief, Paediatric Urology
The Brady Urological Institute
The John Hopkins Hospital
Baltimore, Maryland
USA

Duncan T. Wilcox, MD, FRCS

Associate Professor, Pediatric Urology
The University of Texas Southwestern
Medical Center at Dallas
Dallas, Texas
USA

Blackwell
Publishing

First published 2006

Library of Congress Cataloging-in-Publication Data

Clinical problems in pediatric urology / edited by Prasad Godbole, John P. Gearhart,
    Duncan T. Wilcox.
        p. ; cm.
    Includes bibliographical references.
    ISBN-13: 978-1-4051-2716-5 (alk. paper)
    ISBN-10: 1-4051-2716-3 (alk. paper)
    1. Pediatric urology—Case studies.   2. Pediatric urology—Problems, exercises, etc.   I. Godbole,
Prasad.   II. Gearhart, John P.   III. Wilcox, Duncan T.
    [DNLM: 1. Urologic Diseases—diagnosis—Adolescent—Case Reports.   2. Urologic Diseases—
diagnosis—Adolescent—Problems and Exercises.   3. Urologic Diseases—diagnosis—Child—Case
Reports.   4. Urologic Diseases—diagnosis—Child—Problems and Exercises.   5. Urologic
Diseases—diagnosis—Infant—Case Reports.   6. Urologic Diseases—diagnosis—Infant—Problems
and Exercises.   7. Urogenital Abnormalities—diagnosis—Adolescent—Case Reports.
8. Urogenital Abnormalities—diagnosis—Adolescent—Problems and Exercises.   9. Urogenital
Abnormalities—diagnosis—Child—Case Reports.   10. Urogenital Abnormalities—diagnosis—
Child—Problems and Exercises.   11. Urogenital Abnormalities—diagnosis—Infant—Case Reports.
12. Urogenital Abnormalities—diagnosis—Infant—Problems and Exercises.   13. Urogenital
Abnormalities—therapy—Adolescent—Case Reports.   14. Urogenital Abnormalities—therapy—
Adolescent—Problems and Exercises.   15. Urogenital Abnormalities—therapy—Child—Case
Reports.   16. Urogenital Abnormalities—therapy—Child—Problems and Exercises.
17. Urogenital Abnormalities—therapy—Infant—Case Reports.   18. Urogenital Abnormalities—
therapy—Infant—Problems and Exercises.   19. Urologic Diseases—therapy—Adolescent—Case
Reports.   20. Urologic Diseases—therapy—Adolescent—Problems and Exercises.   21. Urologic
Diseases—therapy—Child—Case Reports.   22. Urologic Diseases—therapy—Child—Problems and
Exercises.   23. Urologic Diseases—therapy—Infant—Case Reports.   24. Urologic
Diseases—therapy—Infant—Problems and Exercises.   WS 18.2 C641 2005]
    RJ466.C54   2005
    618.92′6—dc22

                                                                        2005016404

A catalogue record for this title is available from the British Library

Set in 10/13pt Photina & Frankling Gothic by TechBooks, New Delhi, India
Printed and bound in India by Replika Press PVT Ltd.

Commissioning Editor: Stuart Taylor
Editorial Assistant: Katrina Chandler
Development Editor: Simone Dudziak
Production Controller: Kate Charman

For further information on Blackwell Publishing, visit our website:
http://www.blackwellpublishing.com

The publisher's policy is to use permanent paper from mills that operate a sustainable forestry policy,
and which has been manufactured from pulp processed using acid-free and elementary chlorine-free
practices. Furthermore, the publisher ensures that the text paper and cover board used have met
acceptable environmental accreditation standards.

Contents

Contents

List of Contributors

Laurence S. Baskin, MD
Chief, Pediatric Urology
UCSF Children's Hospital
Professor, Urology and Pediatrics
San Francisco, California
USA

Peter Cuckow, MD, FRCS(Paed)
Consultant Paediatric Urologist
Great Ormond Street Hospital
for Children NHS Trust
London, UK

H. K. Dhillon, FRCS(Edin)
Associate Specialist, Perinatal Urology
Department of Paediatric Urology
Great Ormond Street Hospital for
Children NHS Trust
London, UK

Divyesh. Y. Desai, MD, MS, MCh(Urol)
Paediatric Urologist & Director
Urodynamics Unit
Department of Urology
Great Ormond Street Hospital for
Children NHS Trust
London, UK

Peter C. Fisher, MD
Chief Resident in Urology
University of Michigan Medical School
& Health Center
Ann Arbor, Michigan
USA

Peter D. Furness III, MD
Associate Professor of Surgery
The Children's Hospital
Department of Paediatric Urology
Denver, Colorado
USA

John P. Gearhart, MD, FACS FAAP
Division of Paediatric Urology
Professor & Chief, Paediatric Urology
The Brady Urological Institute
The John Hopkins Hospital
Baltimore, MD
USA

Prasad Godbole, FRCS, FRCS(Paed)
Consultant Paediatric Urologist
Sheffield Children's NHS Trust
Sheffield, UK

Mohan S. Gundeti, MS, MCh(Urol), DNBE(Urol), FEBU
Honorary Specialist Registrar
Great Ormond Street Hospital for
Children
Research Registrar
Guy's & St Thomas Hospital
(Evelina Children's Hospital)
London, UK

Kim A. R. Hutton, MBChB, ChM FRCS(Paed)
Consultant Paediatric Surgeon & Urologist
University Hospital of Wales
Cardiff, UK

Martin Kaefer, MD
Associate Professor, Pediatric Urology
Riley Children's Hospital
Indiana University Medical Center
Indianapolis, Indiana
USA

Martin A. Koyle, MD, FAAP, FACS
Professor of Surgery & Paediatrics
University of Colorado School of Medicine
Denver, Colorado
USA

List of Contributors

A. Ewen MacKinnon, MB, BS, FRCS FRCPCH
Consultant Paediatric Urologist
Department of Paediatric Surgery
Sheffield Children's NHS Trust
Sheffield, UK

Stephen D. Marks, MD, MBChB, MSc, MRCP(UK), DCH, MRCPCH
Consultant Paediatric Nephrologist
Department of Paediatric Nephrology
Great Ormond Street Hospital for
Children NHS Trust
London, UK

Gerald Mingin, MD
Assistant Professor of Surgery & Urology
The University of Colorado
Attending Urologist
The Children's Hospital
Denver, Colorado
USA

Pierre Mouriquand, MD, FRCS(Eng)
Head of the Department of Paediatric
Urology
Debrousse Hospital–Claude-Bernard
University
Lyon, France

Imran Mushtaq, MD, FRCS
Consultant Paediatric Urologist
Department of Paediatric Urology
Great Ormond Street Hospital for
Children NHS Trust
London, UK

Stuart O'Toole, MD, FRCS(Glasg) FRCS(Paeds)
Consultant Paediatric Urologist
Royal Hospital for Sick Children
Glasgow, UK

John M. Park, MD
Associate Professor of Urology
Director, Pediatric Urology
University of Michigan Medical
School & Health Center
Ann Arbor, Michigan
USA

Warren T. Snodgrass, MD
Professor of Urology
Chief, Pediatric Urology
Children's Medical Center Dallas
Dallas, Texas
USA

Hubert S. Swana, MD
Clinical Instructor
Department of Urology
University of California
Children's Medical Center
San Francisco, California
USA

Serdar Tekgül, MD
Chief of Pediatric Urology
Hacettepe University School
of Medicine
Shhiye, Ankara
Turkey

Duncan T. Wilcox, MD, FRCS
Associate Professor, Pediatric Urology
The University of Texas
Southwestern Medical Center at Dallas
Dallas, Texas
USA

Paul Winyard, MD
Senior Lecturer
Nephro-Urology Unit
Institute of Child Health
London, UK

Preface

Pediatric urology as a subspecialty has made rapid progress over the last decade. During this period, medical training has also evolved from a more knowledge-based and factual approach to problem-based learning. Although there are several excellent pediatric urology textbooks available, given the relatively limited number of opportunities available for training in pediatric urology, this textbook discusses the common pediatric urological conditions encountered in clinical practice in a problem-based format.

The aim of this textbook is to help assimilate the factual knowledge obtained into clinical practice and would therefore be useful for trainees in pediatric urology and surgery, adult urology, and adolescent urology as a tool for self assessment, learning, and preparation for examinations. It would be useful to trainers for periodic assessment and validation of their residents. This textbook is not meant to replace the current textbooks, but rather to complement them.

All clinical scenarios in the textbook are from the individual contributors' practice. The clinical scenario is followed by a list of management questions and a discussion regarding the management options. The management for that particular scenario reflects the author's personal practice, but the editors agree that there may be several "correct" options for any given situation. A list of specific, relevant suggested reading is given at the end.

The editors are indebted to the outstanding panel of international contributors for their efforts and outstanding work toward the production of this textbook and in keeping to a very tight deadline. The editors also wish to thank Simone Dudziak and Charlie Hamlyn at Blackwell Publishing for their organization and support for this book from conception to delivery.

And most importantly, a final thank you to all our families, without whose support and sacrifice we would not have been able to dedicate the time and effort required in the publication of this innovative textbook.

Prasad Godbole
John P. Gearhart
Duncan T. Wilcox

1 | Pediatric Nephrology

Stephen D. Marks and Paul Winyard

CASE 1

A male baby is born at 36 weeks' gestation following a diagnosis of bilateral hydroureteronephrosis, thick-walled bladder, and oligohydramnios made at 21 weeks' gestation.

1 What is the most likely underlying diagnosis?

2 What postnatal radiology investigations are required?

3 What investigations will give information about prognosis?

Discussion

1 The most likely underlying diagnosis is posterior urethral valves, which has an estimated incidence of 1 in 5000 to 1 in 8000.

2 The best postnatal radiology investigations are ultrasound of the kidneys and urinary tract (which may show a thick-walled, poorly emptying bladder with upper tract dilatation and possible aberrant kidney development) and micturating cystourethrogram.

3 The best prognostic indicators are the size of kidneys, amount of renal parenchyma, and corticomedullary differentiation. Other prognostic indicators are plasma creatinine at 1 month of age, measured glomerular filtration rate (e.g. using 51-labeled chromium EDTA) at 12 months of age, and later formal urodynamic assessment.

Consider the same case, but with placement of vesicoamniotic shunt at 31 weeks, which appeared to work initially (i.e. led to reduced dilatation) but was then lost and presumed to be dislodged. What is the likely cause of a rapidly rising urea and creatinine within a few days after birth?

This may reflect the underlying severe renal disease but might also represent occult internalization of shunt, which can drain into the peritoneal cavity generating urinary ascites, which is reabsorbed and exacerbates apparent renal dysfunction.

Suggested reading

Duffy PG. Posterior urethral valves and other urethral abnormalities. In: Thomas DFM, Rickwood AMK, Duffy PG, eds. *Essentials of Pediatric Urology*. London, UK: Martin Dunitz; 2002:87–96.

Mesrobian HG, Balcom AH, Durkee CT. Urologic problems of the neonate. *Pediatr Clin North Am.* 2004;51(4):1051–62.

Schober JM, Dulabon LM, Woodhouse CR. Outcome of valve ablation in late-presenting posterior urethral valves. *BJU Int.* 2004;94(4):616–19.

Strand WR. Initial management of complex pediatric disorders: prune belly syndrome, posterior urethral valves. *Urol Clin North Am.* 2004;31(3):399–415.

Ylinen E, Ala-Houhala M, Wikstrom S. Prognostic factors of posterior urethral valves and the role of antenatal detection. *Pediatr Nephrol.* 2004;19(8):874–9.

CASE 2

A term baby girl, who was born weighing 3 kg, is admitted to the pediatric intensive care unit at 14 days of age. She is breastfeeding reasonably and has continuous wet nappies. On examination, she weighs 2.4 kg and appears dehydrated and unwell. Her observations reveal systolic blood pressure of 40 mm Hg. Investigations show the following values: hemoglobin, 19 g/dl; WBC count, 12×10^9/l; platelet count, 246×10^9/l; sodium, 125 mmol/l; potassium, 6.5 mmol/l; urea, 10.4mmol/l; and plasma creatinine, 250μmol/l. Abdominal ultrasound shows a provisional diagnosis of bilateral renal dysplasia and bilateral pelviureteric junction (PUJ) obstruction.

1 What immediate management would you institute?

2 What other urgent tests are required?

3 When she is better and tolerating enteral feeds, what further management might she require?

Discussion

1 Although initially term babies can lose up to 10% of their birth weight, they usually regain this by day 10. However, this baby has lost 20% of her birth weight at 2 weeks of age, and clinically this represents severe dehydration. The immediate management would be confirmation of hypovolemic shock looking for prolonged capillary refill time and other signs of poor peripheral perfusion. She required urgent resuscitation with a bolus of 20 ml/kg of crystalloid (such as 0.9% sodium chloride) and commencement of intravenous broad-spectrum antibiotics, ideally after samples of urine, blood, and cerebrospinal fluid for culture and sensitivity.

2 Other urgent tests required are blood gas with tCO2, serum glucose, calcium, and phosphate.

3 As she improves, the urinary tract ultrasound should be repeated, as initial ultrasound when neonates are dehydrated may not show definitive pathologies and true size of dilatation. Long-term prophylactic antibiotics must also be considered. Many children with renal dysplasia are obligate salt losers (with consistently high urinary sodium levels of 60–80 mmol/l), polyuric (even when dehydrated), and also usually quite acidotic. They may require large quantities of both sodium chloride and sodium bicarbonate to correct these losses, first intravenously and then enterally. Long-term supplementation with sodium chloride and sodium bicarbonate will also be required, but take care not to overdo it when requirements fall as the renal function deteriorates.

Suggested reading

Cuckow PM, Nyirady P, Winyard PJ. Normal and abnormal development of the urogenital tract. *Prenat Diagn.* 2001;21(11):908–916.

Mackway-Jones K, Molyneux E, Phillips B, Wieteska S. *Advanced Paediatric Life Support. The Practical Approach.* 3rd ed. London, UK: Advanced Life Support Group and British Medical Journal Books.

Piscione TD, Rosenblum ND. The molecular control of renal branching morphogenesis: current knowledge and emerging insights. *Differentiation.* 2002;70(6):227–46.

Winyard PJD, Chitty L. Dysplastic and polycystic kidneys: diagnosis, associations and management. *Prenat Diagn.* 2001;21(11):924–35.

Woolf AS, Price KL, Scambler PJ, Winyard PJD. Evolving concepts in human renal dysplasia. *J Am Soc Nephrol.* 2004;15(4):998–1007.

CASE 3

A female baby who is the third child of healthy, nonconsanguinous parents is born with hydrops fetalis at 34 weeks' gestation and weighs 2.5 kg. There was evidence of polyhydramnios, and antenatal diagnosis at 24 weeks' gestation revealed bilateral hydroureteronephrosis (with left renal pelvis measuring $1.5 \times 2 \times 3$ cm, and right renal pelvis measuring $1.5 \times 1.5 \times 2.5$ cm). She developed bilateral pleural effusions at 28 weeks' gestation, which required insertion of a right-sided shunt at 32 weeks' gestation (by which time the left kidney was noted to be duplex, with the left renal pelvis measuring $4 \times 2.5 \times 4.5$ cm and the right renal pelvis measuring $3 \times 3.5 \times 5.5$ cm).

Postnatally, she was noted to be dysmorphic with bilateral cataracts, low-set ears, and microcephaly. She had bilateral pleural effusions, which required insertion of left chest drain and high-frequency ventilation.

Despite insertion of a suprapubic catheter, which remained unobstructed, she developed acute oligoanuric renal failure and abdominal distension with increasing ascites, and her repeat renal ultrasound revealed evidence of increasing dilatation with both renal pelves measuring 2.5 cm.

1 What intervention is now required?

2 What investigations are required to work out a unifying diagnosis?

3 What radiology investigations are required?

Discussion

1 This child clearly has bilateral renal obstruction, which requires immediate drainage with insertion of bilateral nephrostomies.

2 The two most likely causes of this clinical situation are chromosomal abnormalities and congenital infections. Therefore, investigations should include karyotype or chromosomal analysis (with another specimen to save DNA for further analysis in case specific syndromes are queried later) and congenital infection screen for parvovirus and TORCH infections (e.g. toxoplasmosis, rubella, cytomegalovirus, hepatitis).

3 Radiology investigations should include repeat renal ultrasounds, bilateral nephrostograms, cranial ultrasound, and echocardiography.

After relief of the obstruction, her urine output improves with polyuria but the creatinine remains elevated and only comes down to a minimum value of 450 μmol/l. On repeat renal ultrasound, there is only a thin rim of renal parenchyma bilaterally. What is the prognosis, and what options should be discussed with the family and the multidisciplinary team? If she survives, what are the most important issues for her first year of life?

- The prognosis is bleak; with these results it is almost inevitable that she will require early renal replacement therapy for survival.
- The options that may be discussed with her parents are as follows:
  1 *Medical management to optimize nutrition and growth.* This will involve close monitoring and treatment of anemia; calcium, phosphate, and PTH levels; and acid/base and fluid status. Supplemental nutrition will require nasogastric or gastrostomy feeding.
  2 *Surgery to ensure adequate drainage of her collecting systems.* Prophylactic antibiotics should also be prescribed.
  3 *Renal replacement therapy.* Peritoneal dialysis may be difficult in view of the ascites, and hemodialysis would be technically more difficult due to her prematurity and size. If possible, the aim would be to avoid these and maximize growth and weight gain (as seen above), since renal transplantation becomes technically easier as children approach 10 kg.

4 *Minimal treatment.* Although it is contentious, some centers will discuss the option not to treat her aggressively, since she has involvement of many systems and treatment may prolong lifespan but not improve her quality of life.

Suggested reading

Clark TJ, Martin WL, Divakaran TG, Whittle MJ, Kilby MD, Khan KS. Prenatal bladder drainage in the management of fetal lower urinary tract obstruction: a systematic review and meta-analysis. *Obstet Gynecol.* 2003;102(2):367–82.

Favre R, Dreux S, Dommergues M, et al. Nonimmune fetal ascites: a series of 79 cases. *Am J Obstet Gynecol.* 2004;190(2):407–12.

Newton ER. Diagnosis of perinatal TORCH infections. *Clin Obstet Gynecol.* 1999;42(1):59–70.

Shooter M, Watson A. The ethics of withholding and withdrawing dialysis therapy in infants. *Pediatr Nephrol.* Apr 2000;14(4):347–51.

Skoll MA, Sharland GK, Allan LD. Is the ultrasound definition of fluid collections in non-immune hydrops fetalis helpful in defining the underlying cause or predicting outcome? *Ultrasound Obstet Gynecol.* 1991;1(5):309–12.

CASE 4

A 14-year-old boy had a cadaveric renal transplantation 12 years ago for end-stage renal failure secondary to posterior urethral valves, bilateral renal dysplasia, and bilateral vesicoureteric reflux. He is admitted for bladder augmentation with ileocystoplasty, ureteric reimplantation, and Mitrofanoff formation. His medications are alternate-day prednisolone, azathioprine, ciclosporin, amlodipine, ferrous sulphate, and 1-alpha-hydroxycholecalciferol. His last measured glomerular filtration rate was 30 ml/min/ 1.73 m^2.

1 What blood tests should he have preoperatively?

2 Name two blood tests that are so important preoperatively that their results may delay surgery.

3 What is the most important aspect of his preoperative clinical examination?

4 How much fluid should be given preoperatively?

5 Perioperatively and postoperatively, what medications need to be given and what monitoring should be given?

6 What are the risks of this operation to his renal function that should be discussed during consent?

Discussion

1 The standard preoperative investigations for a patient undergoing this surgery should include the following:
   - Full blood count, coagulation screen, cross-match 4 units.
   - Serum electrolytes (Na, K, Cl, tCO_2, urea, creatinine), liver function.
   As this patient has chronic renal failure and has had a renal transplant further investigations should include:
   - Ferritin (as he may have iron deficiency).
   - Bone profile with ionized calcium and PTH (chronic renal failure of this magnitude is normally associated with secondary hyperparathyroidism, which if untreated or undertreated, e.g. if there is poor adherence to his 1-alpha-hydroxycholecalciferol medication, may result in hypocalcaemia).
   - Trough ciclosporin level (to ensure that there is adequate immunosuppression preoperatively as this may need to be given intravenously postoperatively).
2 Results that should be particularly noted preoperatively include the following:
   - Hemoglobin (should increase his hemoglobin with Erythropoeitin prior to surgery).
   - Creatinine level (if this has increased preoperatively, then surgery should be delayed until the cause is found).
   - Other results that may prevent surgery taking place, e.g. hypocalcemia (see above), hyperkalemia, acidosis, hyponatremia, hypernatremia, etc.
3 The most important aspect of his preoperative clinical examination is measurement of his blood pressure, as he is on antihypertensive treatment with amlodipine and may have poor control.
4 To ascertain how much fluid should be given preoperatively, ask for his 24-hour fluid target and divide this by 24 to give the rate in milliliters per hour of infusion of 0.45% sodium chloride and 2.5% dextrose to be commenced when nil by mouth. Postoperatively, he may require more fluids due to additional losses.
5 Perioperatively and postoperatively, the following need to be given:
   - Intravenous antibiotic cover with dosages adjusted for renal failure and trough level results should be known prior to further doses of nephrotoxic antibiotics (such as amikacin, gentamicin, or vancomycin).
   - Intravenous immunosuppression to prevent rejection.
   - Careful postoperative monitoring of his blood pressure to maintain renal perfusion. Antihypertensive medications may be required postoperatively for severe hypertension. Agents such as intravenous hydralazine

could be given when nil by mouth. Care should be taken to maintain normal blood pressure and avoid episodes of hypertension and hypotension.

6 The risks of this operation include deterioration of renal function with the risk of acute or chronic renal failure due to acute tubular necrosis from hypovolemia, hypoxia, and nephrotoxicity with antibiotics and immunosuppression. Because he was transplanted at a young age and probably had an intra-abdominal transplant, there is an increased risk of direct surgical complications to the transplanted kidney.

Suggested reading

Avner ED, Harmon WE, Niaudet P. *Pediatric Nephrology*. 5th ed. Philadelphia: Lippincott; 2004:1267–1478.

DeFoor W, Tackett L, Minevich E, et al. Successful renal transplantation in children with posterior urethral valves. *J Urol*. 2003;170(6):2402–4.

Koo HP, Bunchman TE, Flynn JT, Punch JD, Schwartz AC, Bloom DA. Renal transplantation in children with severe lower urinary tract dysfunction. *J Urol*. 1999;161(1):240–5.

Luke PP, Herz DB, Bellinger MF, et al. Long-term results of pediatric renal transplantation into a dysfunctional lower urinary tract. *Transplantation*. 2003;76(11):1578–82.

Rigden SPA. The management of chronic and end stage renal failure in children. In: Webb NJA, Postlethwaite RJ, ed. *Clinical Paediatric Nephrology*. 3rd ed. Oxford, UK: Oxford University Press; 2003:427–45.

CASE 5

A 5-year-old girl with VACTERL association had a live-related renal transplantation from her father 15 months ago. She had chronic renal failure secondary to a right nonfunctioning multicystic kidney and a lower lying left cystic kidney, with no ureter draining the upper moiety and an atretic ureter from the left lower moiety. She previously had multiple urological and general surgical procedures including percutaneous JJ stent insertion between her lower ureter and bladder, reimplantation of her native ureter, right nephrectomy and colostomy formation for her imperforate anus, and posterior sagittal anorectoplasty, with closure of colostomy. She has a variant of cloacal dysgenesis and urogenital sinus and has thoracic scoliosis as part of her VACTERL association.

Her posttransplantation plasma creatinine levels were 17–20 µmol/l. Six months post transplantation, she underwent bladder neck reconstruction with ileocystoplasty and formation of her Mitrofanoff channel. However, postoperatively her creatinine increased from 36 to 58 µmol/l, and 2 months later, this had not returned to its baseline.

1 What could be the causes for her increased creatinine?

2 What investigations should you consider to help make the diagnosis?

Discussion

1 Her increased creatinine perioperatively may be due to acute factors such as dehydration, obstruction and poor drainage, acute rejection, and infections, particularly urinary tract infections. Since the creatinine has stayed elevated, additional longer-term factors need to be considered, such as chronic allograft nephropathy, toxicity from her calcineurin inhibitors as part of her immunosuppression (ciclosporin or tacrolimus toxicity), and renal artery stenosis; all of these are likely to be associated with elevated blood pressure. In addition, check for intercurrent infections such as Epstein Barr virus, cytomegalovirus, and bacterial and other infections.

2 Further investigations should include accurate fluid status from history and clinical examination, drug levels, abdominal ultrasound (including Doppler transplant renal ultrasound with bladder residuals), and DTPA scan. More invasive investigations, pending the above results, might include transplant renal biopsy, antegrade pyelography, and formal urodynamics.

Suggested reading

Kerr B, Webb NJA. Renal malformations and renal involvement in syndromes. In: Webb NJA, Postlethwaite RJ, eds. *Clinical Paediatric Nephrology*. 3rd ed. Oxford, UK: Oxford University Press; 2003:317–28.

Nankivell BJ, Borrows RJ, Fung CL, O'Connell PJ, Chapman JR, Allen RD. Calcineurin inhibitor nephrotoxicity: longitudinal assessment by protocol histology. *Transplantation*. 2004;78(4):557–65.

Patankar JZ, Vidyadhar M, Prabhakaran K, Bo L, Lsk Loh D. Urogenital sinus, rectovaginal fistula, and an anterior stenosed anus – another cloacal variant. *Pediatr Surg Int*. 2004;20(7):556–8.

Thomas DFM. Cystic renal disease. In: Thomas DFM, Rickwood AMK, Duffy PG, eds. *Essentials of Pediatric Urology*. London, UK: Martin Dunitz; 2002:97–104.

2 | Perinatal Urology

H. K. Dhillon

CASE 1

A 3-day-old baby boy has had an ultrasound following a prenatal diagnosis of left hydronephrosis. The ultrasound appearances of the left kidney are shown below.

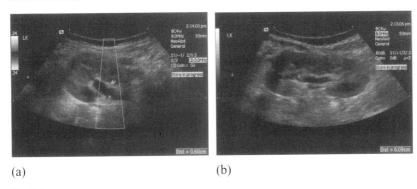

(a)   (b)

Fig. 2.1

1 How would you describe the degree of dilatation of the pelvicalyceal system?
2 How would you manage this child?
3 Would you recommend that this baby be maintained on prophylaxis?
4 What is the natural history of this degree of dilatation?

Discussion

1 At 6 mm this dilatation is mild (<15 mm) and there is no calyceal involvement.
2 The management of prenatally diagnosed abnormalities demands documentation of the prenatal findings so that subsequent management is not solely dependent on the first postnatal ultrasound. The optimal management of a "mild" dilatation is dependent more on the prenatal findings than any other degree of renal pelvic dilatation. The term *mild dilatation* should be reserved for cases where the dilatation does not exceed 15 mm in the third trimester and where there is no calyceal or ureteric dilatation.

A postnatal mild dilatation may be an artifact (as in Case 2) and mislead the clinician into managing a baby with a severe pelviureteric junction (PUJ) obstruction conservatively. A postnatal unilateral mild dilatation could also be an artifact masking severe vesicoureteric reflux. In such cases the prenatal findings would have demonstrated abnormalities that would justify a micturating cysturethrogram (MCUG).

The prenatal findings for this baby were as follows:
- 20 weeks' gestation – Two normal kidneys. Normal bladder and amniotic fluid.
- 34 weeks' gestation (routine ultrasound) – Left renal pelvis measured 7 mm. No calyceal dilatation. Right kidney, bladder, and amniotic fluid normal.

The prenatal history with a dilatation of only 7 mm appearing late in pregnancy clarifies that the right kidney does not have a PUJ abnormality. This is a mild upper tract late third trimester dilatation.

The next investigation for this baby would be a further ultrasound at 3 months of age, and this could be repeated at 1 year of age. Routine cystography for children with this degree of dilatation is commonplace and unjustified. The only absolute indications for a MCUG are pre- or postnatal abnormalities of the bladder, ureteric dilatation, bilateral hydronephroses, and duplex kidney(s). Unselected cystography for infants with prenatal hydronephrosis will reveal reflux in less than 15% of cases. Approximately half of these will have reflux associated with a pre- and postnatal unilateral mild pelvic dilatation. The reflux in these cases will be either grade 2 or grade 3 into two normally functioning kidneys. Children with reflux into two normal kidneys on a DMSA scan will have stopped refluxing by 15 months of age. The majority of these patients are male and historically did not present clinically. The apparent association between severe reflux and a postnatal mild dilatation is a consequence of ignoring the prenatal findings. The prenatal histories would have identified a dilated ureter or ureters, bilateral hydronephroses, or an abnormal bladder. A more preferable option to routine cystography would be to advise the parents to ensure that a urine specimen is tested if the child is unwell. Further investigations such as a MCUG should only be recommended if the child had a symptomatic urinary tract infection. Some pediatric units have adopted the alternative policy of maintaining children with a mild dilatation on prophylaxis for the first year of life.

Children with a pre- and postnatal mild unilateral dilatation and normal calyces do not require a radioisotope study.

3 Infants with a mild dilatation who do not fulfill the pre- and postnatal criteria for an MCUG do not require prophylaxis.

4 Mild dilatations either resolve spontaneously or remain stable. There is no current evidence to suggest that unilateral pre- and postnatal mild dilatation without calyceal involvement can progress to a PUJ obstruction, which requires surgery. Routine cystography is inappropriate as a means of ensuring that severe reflux is not missed, as the prenatal history will identify the population at risk.

CASE 2

A 4-day-old baby boy has had an ultrasound following a prenatal diagnosis of left hydronephrosis. The baby is perfectly well and was started on trimethoprim prophylaxis on the first day of life. The ultrasound appearances of the left kidney are as shown.

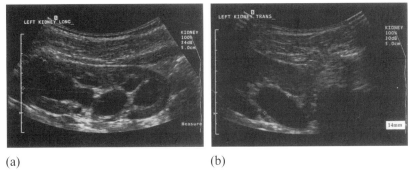

(a)   (b)

Fig. 2.2

1 How would you describe the degree of dilatation of the pelvicalyceal system?
2 How would you manage this baby?
3 What would be the indications for surgery?

Discussion

1 This dilatation measures 14 mm, which is within the category of "mild" dilatation. However, there is severe calyceal dilatation, and a discrepancy between the degree of pelvic and calyceal dilatation usually arises because the ultrasound was carried out while the baby was not well hydrated or after it had emptied its bladder. Thus the state of the bladder on the ultrasound, as well as the degree of pelvicalyceal dilatation, has to be considered. The other explanation for this appearance is that this is an intrarenal variety of hydronephrosis where the renal pelvis usually measures less than 15 mm but the calyces are as or even more dilated than the renal pelvis.

2 The prenatal history will clarify whether the pelvis is more dilated than the postnatal scan suggests and also whether the dilatation had increased prenatally:

- 20 weeks' gestation – Left renal pelvis measured 14 mm with mild calyceal dilatation. Normal right kidney, bladder, and amniotic fluid.
- 28 weeks' gestation – Left hydronephrosis of 22 mm with calyceal dilatation. No other abnormality of the renal tract. Amniotic fluid normal.
- 36 weeks' gestation – Left renal pelvis 33 mm with severe calyceal dilatation. No other abnormality noted.

The prenatal history identifies this child as having a severe left hydronephrosis, which has increased progressively and can only be caused by an abnormality at the PUJ. The first postnatal ultrasound was an artifact and highlights the need to base management on the prenatal findings.

The prenatal history clarifies that the first postnatal investigation after the preliminary ultrasound should be a repeat ultrasound and radioisotope study (MAG3) as close to 1 month of age as possible. Four to 6 weeks of age would be an ideal time for such a study.

3 The indications for pyeloplasty in infants with severe hydronephrosis are reduced function (<40%) either at the outset or later and increasing dilatation or symptoms. A baby with a history of progressive dilatation of the renal pelvis with calyceal dilatation that exceeds 30 mm in the third trimester will either have reduced function at the outset or will have a more than 75% chance of subsequently deteriorating from initial good function. Conservative management for infants with initial good function will involve close follow-up with further ultrasounds and radioisotope studies at 3–6-month intervals. This population will therefore benefit from pyeloplasty in the first 6 months of life as the high risk of functional deterioration, as well as the radiation burden, does not justify conservative management. Post-Lasix drainage curves will be "obstructed" in this high-risk group. However, most hydronephroses of more than 15 mm with calyceal dilatation will also drain poorly under the influence of a diuretic load. The majority of this population with 15–30-mm hydronephroses have not required surgery and are either stable or have improved spontaneously.

CASE 3

A 3-day-old baby girl has had an ultrasound following a prenatal diagnosis of right hydronephrosis. The ultrasound appearances of the kidney are as shown below.

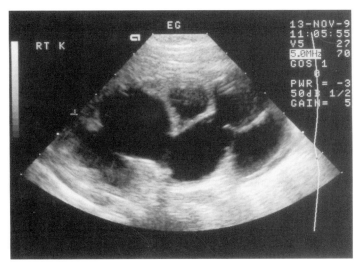

Fig. 2.3

1 How would you describe this degree of dilatation of the pelvicalyceal system?

2 How would you manage this baby? What would be the indications for surgery for this degree of pelvicalyceal dilatation?

Discussion

1 The dilatation measures 12 mm, but there is severe calyceal dilatation. The prenatal findings were as follows:
  - 20 weeks' gestation – Mild right hydronephrosis (7 mm). Normal left kidney, bladder, and amniotic fluid.
  - 34 weeks' gestation – Right multicystic kidney? Hydronephrosis? Normal left kidney, bladder, and amniotic fluid.

The prenatal history of mild dilatation and an uncertainty about whether the kidney is multicystic should raise the suspicion that this is an intrarenal type of hydronephrosis.

2 Intrarenal hydronephroses are atypical in that the renal pelvis may be mildly dilated but the calyces are clubbed and may be more dilated than the renal pelvis. This type of hydronephrosis is difficult to manage conservatively as the kidney function can change without any increase in the size of the renal pelvis. The clearance image on the radioisotope study will show severe defects in the parenchyma caused by the dilated calyces. Conservative management will require close follow-up and repeat radioisotope studies at 3–6-month intervals. This population is an exception and should not be followed on the basis of the degree of renal pelvic dilatation alone. Children with an intrarenal variety of hydronephrosis and good function justify a pyeloplasty by 6 months of age. This can lead to considerable improvement in the appearances of the parenchyma. Figures 2.4a and 2.4b show the pre- and postoperative MAG3 studies of the kidney shown in Fig. 2.3.

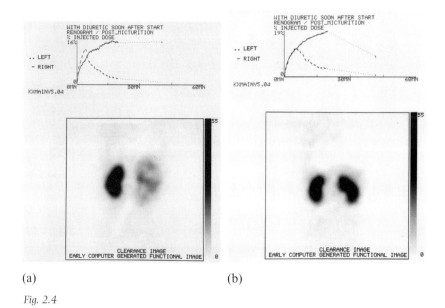

(a)   (b)

Fig. 2.4

CASE 4

A three-day-old baby boy has had an ultrasound showing a bilateral dilatation of both his kidneys. The ultrasound appearances are as shown below.

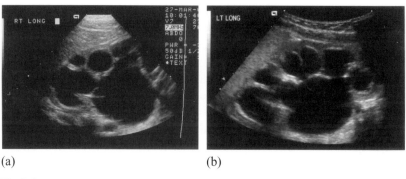

(a)   (b)

Fig. 2.5

1 How would you describe the degree of dilatation of the pelvicalyceal systems?
2 How would you manage this baby?
3 What would be the indications for surgery with these findings?

Discussion

1 This baby has bilateral severe dilatation of the renal pelves and calyces. A male baby with these findings could either have a bilateral problem at the PUJ or a lower urinary tract anomaly.
2 The prenatal history will clarify whether this is an upper or lower tract anomaly. The prenatal history is as follows:
   - 20 weeks' gestation – Right kidney 10 mm pelvis, left kidney 12 mm pelvis. Normal bladder and amniotic fluid.
   - 28 weeks' gestation – Right kidney 18 mm pelvis with calyceal dilatation, left kidney 20 mm with calyceal dilatation. Normal bladder and amniotic fluid.
   - 34 weeks' gestation – Right kidney 22 mm pelvis with calyceal dilatation, left kidney 26 mm with calyceal dilatation. Normal bladder and amniotic fluid. Ureters not visualized.

   Male infants with bilateral hydronephroses routinely have an MCUG as part of their management. The prenatal history of this baby clarifies that there was no lower urinary tract problem, and this baby is extremely unlikely to have a urethral obstruction. In the absence of a good prenatal history it would still be justifiable to proceed with an early cystogram to ensure that urethral abnormalities are not missed. This baby will require a radioisotope study at about 4–6 weeks of age, and cystography should be timed so as not to cause any delay in assessing the individual kidney function.
3 Children with a severe bilateral upper tract dilatation (>20 mm with calyceal clubbing) or a severe dilatation in a solitary kidney should not be managed conservatively as this risks deterioration of their overall renal function. The first radioisotope study will either show two equally functioning kidneys (which may actually have similarly reduced function) or one kidney with reduced function. Pyeloplasty would be advisable for the severely hydronephrotic kidney with reduced function provided that there was more than 15% uptake. In the presence of one very poorly functioning kidney it would be more logical to proceed with pyeloplasty for the severely hydronephrotic side with better function. The poorly functioning kidney could have a pigtail catheter inserted at the same time to clarify if there

is any salvageable function. In cases where both kidneys are functioning equally, the side with the greater degree of hydronephrosis should have a pyeloplasty by 3 months of age. The second side will require close follow-up at 3-month intervals. Any concern regarding the degree of dilatation or function would warrant a contralateral pyeloplasty. Children who have had a unilateral pyeloplasty and still have a severe stable contralateral dilatation should have a formal estimation of their glomerular filtration rate (GFR) after 1 year of age. Continuing conservative management would only be justified if the GFR was normal.

Suggested reading

Dhillon HK. Prenatally diagnosed hydronephrosis: the Great Ormond Street experience. *Br J Urol.* 1998;81(suppl 2):39–44.

Dhillon HK. Prenatal diagnosis. In: Thomas DFM, Rickwood AMK, Duffy PG, eds. *Essentials of Paediatric Urology.* London, UK: Martin Dunitz; 2002:97–104.

Feldman DM, DeCambre M, Kong E, et al. Evaluation and follow-up of fetal hydronephrosis. *J Ultrasound Med.* Oct 2001;20(10):1065–9.

Godley ML, Desai D, Yeung CK, Dhillon HK, Duffy PG, Ransley PG. The relationship between early renal status and the resolution of vesico-ureteric reflux and bladder function at 16 months. *Br J Urol Int.* 2001;87:457–62.

Gordon I. Diuretic renography in infants with prenatal unilateral hydronephrosis: an explanation for the controversy about poor drainage. *BJU Int.* Apr 2001;87(6):551–5.

Ransley PG, Dhillon HK, Gordon I, Duffy PG, Dillon MJ, Barratt TM. The postnatal management of hydronephrosis diagnosed by prenatal ultrasound. *J Urol.* 1990;144:584–7.

Thomas DF, Madden NP, Irving HC, Arthur RJ, Smith SE. Mild dilatation of the fetal kidney: a follow-up study. *Br J Urol.* 1994;74(2):236–9.

Ulman I, Jayanthi VR, Koff SA. The long-term followup of newborns with severe unilateral hydronephrosis initially treated non-operatively. *J Urol.* 2000;164(3 pt 2):1101–5.

Yeung CK, Godley ML, Dhillon HK, Gordon I, Duffy PG, Ransley PG. The characteristics of primary vesico-ureteric reflux in male and female infants with prenatal hydronephrosis. *Br J Urol.* Apr 1997;80:319–27.

CASE 5

A fetal ultrasound at 34/40 weeks' gestation shows an abnormality of one kidney (Fig. 2.6).

1 How would you describe the appearances of the kidney?

2 What would be the next investigation for this baby?

3 Would you maintain this baby on prophylactic antibiotics?
4 What is the natural history of such kidneys?
5 What are the indications for surgery?

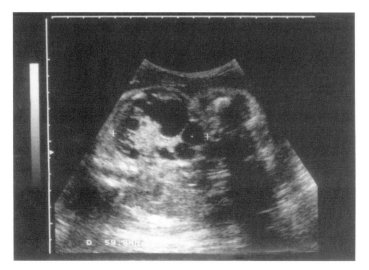

Fig. 2.6

Discussion

1 The appearances are typical of a multicystic dysplastic kidney (MCDK) with cysts of varying sizes that do not communicate. No dilated pelvis is seen, and there is solid tissue centrally.

2 The next investigation will depend on the prenatal history, which is as follows:

- 20 weeks' gestation – Left multicystic kidney, 4 cm. Normal right kidney, bladder, and amniotic fluid.
- 32 weeks' gestation – Left multicystic kidney, 4 cm. Normal right kidney, bladder, and amniotic fluid.

The timing and choice of investigations in this population are dictated by the contralateral rather than the multicystic kidney. This baby has a solitary functioning right kidney with no dilatation pre- and postnatally and a normal lower urinary tract. Postnatal investigations should be geared toward confirming that the right kidney is entirely normal.

The next investigation for this baby should be a further ultrasound and radioisotope study at about 3 months of age. This could be a DMSA scan or a MAG3 if a good clearance image can be obtained. Follow-up after that should be minimal. A further ultrasound at 1 year of age will suffice.

Children with no other detected abnormality of the urinary tract do not routinely require an MCUG. Routine cystography will identify up to 20% of contralateral or ipsilateral reflux. The reflux is usually distal without dilatation of the ureter and pelvicalyceal system and will resolve spontaneously. An MCUG should be reserved for children with a prenatally diagnosed multicystic kidney, with ultrasound evidence of an abnormal bladder or dilatation of the contralateral kidney or ureter. An infant who does not fulfill the criteria for cystography and presents with a symptomatic urinary tract infection will usually require an MCUG.

Children with a prenatally diagnosed multicystic kidney benefit from a formal estimation of their (GFR) after 1 year of age. This will allow those with a normal GFR to be discharged, while those with unpredictable reduced function can be referred for nephrological follow-up.

3 Prophylaxis is required for children who warrant an MCUG, as well as for those who may have a contralateral obstruction at the pelvi- or vesicoureteric junction. The prophylaxis should be discontinued if reflux is not detected and the dilatation is mild. Children with a dilatation of the contralateral kidney associated with calyceal clubbing will require close follow-up with a low threshold for recommending pyeloplasty if the dilatation increases or was severe from the outset. Similarly, hydronephrosis with a very dilated ureter may require intervention for an obstruction at the vesicoureteric junction.

4 The natural history of multicystic kidneys is one of involution that can occur prenatally but is more usual over the first few years. Almost 50% of MCDKs will be difficult to detect on ultrasound by 5 years of age.

There are very few indications for a nephrectomy in the multicystic population. In a few instances the multicystic kidney is so large and easily visible that it will benefit from removal in the first few months. Similarly, multicystic kidneys that are not visible as an abdominal mass but remain large (usually more than 7–8 cm in length) could be removed to simplify follow-up and any potential for injury. Multicystic kidneys with an ipsilateral abnormality (dilated distal ureter, ureterocoele) may also benefit form nephrectomy as the presence of a nonfunctioning kidney and distal dilatation may predispose to infections. The decision to recommend nephrectomy on the basis of the potential risk of hypertension or tumor remains controversial. The risk of hypertension is less than 0.1%, while that of malignant change has been estimated at 1: 2500. Therefore, currently there is insufficient evidence to justify prophylactic nephrectomy.

Children who are discharged without nephrectomy would benefit from having their blood pressure recorded at approximately 1-year intervals.

Suggested reading

Manzoni GM, Caldamone AA. Multicystic kidney. In: Stringer MD, Oldham KT, Mouriquand PDE, Howard ER, eds. *Paediatric Surgery and Urology: Long Term Outcome.* London, UK: Saunders; 1998:632–41.

Thomas DFM. Cystic renal disease. In: Rickwood AMK, Duffy PG, eds. *Essentials of Paediatric Urology.* London, UK: Martin Dunitz; 2002:97–104.

3 | Urodynamics

Divyesh Y. Desai

Introduction

The objective of urodynamic assessments in children is to reproduce their complaints or symptoms (e.g. wetting) and, following the assessment, contribute a pathophysiological explanation for the problem.

A full evaluation will define the pressure/volume relationships within the container in order to ascertain whether the bladder storage is low pressure and thus safe. The assessment would also try to determine if there are any abnormal dynamics that could potentially be detrimental to renal function, which may be treated in order to reduce morbidity.

A more specialist application of pediatric urodynamics is to understand the evolving natural history of lower urinary tract function in specific pathological conditions such as posterior urethral valves and vesicoureteric reflux.

A poor understanding and inappropriate management of lower urinary tract function can result in impaired renal function and unnecessary morbidity, which can handicap a child for life.

Any method that measures function or dysfunction of the lower urinary tract constitutes a urodynamic investigation. Broadly the investigations can be classified into two groups:

1 simple or noninvasive urodynamics;
2 formal or invasive urodynamics.

Simple urodynamics

These assessments are performed in all children referred for evaluation. Following this initial assessment, some children will go on to have a formal invasive urodynamic study.

Frequency/volume diary. In children who are toilet trained, the diary is extremely useful in providing information regarding the nature of the problem in the child's home environment. This is compared with the clinical assessments that are performed in an environment that is new to the child and can influence the results. The diary documents the periodicity and volumes of bladder emptying during the day and gives an idea about the functional bladder capacity in the daytime; the first void in the morning usually reflects the maximum bladder capacity.

Furthermore, the diary can act as a positive feedback tool and a yardstick to assess the efficacy of treatment.

Interview. In addition to obtaining a good medical history, the time spent with the child and family helps to evaluate the child's nature and attitude to the problem being assessed, obtain information regarding the child's home and school environment, and assess the child's compliance for proposed interventions.

Bladder function assessment. This involves at least two free voids into a uroflowmeter, observation of the child's posture during micturition noting whether there is any abdominal effort during voiding, postmicturition dribbling, and postvoid residual urine assessment using ultrasound.

Formal or invasive urodynamics

The various types of formal studies include:
1 standard artificial filling cystometrogram;
2 video contrast filling cystometrogram;
3 isotope filling cystometrogram;
4 natural filling urodynamics.
The three commonly used studies are the natural fill, standard artificial fill, and video contrast fill studies.

These studies are performed via a single- or double-lumen suprapubic catheter, which is placed in the patient under anesthesia at least 24 hours prior to the study. If the storage dynamics are the only aspect to be studied, then these can be assessed via a urethral catheter when children do not have urethral sensation. Abdominal pressure is recorded via a rectal catheter, and pelvic floor/sphincter activity can be recorded using surface or needle electrodes, although the latter is rarely undertaken.

CASE 1

A 6-month-old girl with covered spinal dysraphism and spinal cord tethering was routinely reviewed following spinal cord untethering at 3 months of age.

Pre-untethering ultrasonography of the urinary tract showed two normal kidneys. Post-untethering bladder function assessment showed incomplete bladder emptying; she was commenced on intermittent catheterization twice a day. She had one urinary tract infection, and a follow-up ultrasound scan

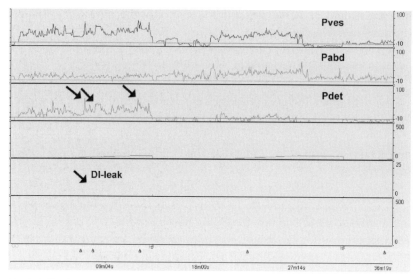

Fig. 3.1 Urodynamic trace pre Oxybutinin.

showed left hydroureteronephrosis and a thick-walled bladder. In view of these findings a micturating cystourethrogram and a DMSA were arranged along with urodynamic studies.

The micturating cystourethrogram showed the bladder holding 20 ml of contrast; the bladder then emptied spontaneously, and during voiding there was a left vesicoureteric reflux grade 2. The DMSA scan showed the right kidney to be normal and contributing 65% to overall renal function. The left kidney was smaller with globally reduced uptake and contributed 35% to overall renal function.

On natural filling urodynamics in the filling phase, there was instability from very early on during filling: 20 ml, with pressure rises of 30–50 cm of water associated with leakage. The compliance was reduced following the instability (Fig. 3.1). In view of these findings she was started on Oxybutinin 1.25 mg twice a day, with intermittent catheterization increased to 4 times a day. On this regime, she was clinically well and developed dry intervals of between 1.5 and 2 hours. Volumes obtained on intermittent catheterization were approximately 150 ml. She was constipated, requiring Sennakot and lactulose with glycerin suppositories to maintain regular bowel emptying.

A follow-up ultrasound scan 3 months later showed an increase in the left hydroureteronephrosis and dilatation of the right lower ureter, which was a new finding. Repeat urodynamic studies were arranged, and the trace is illustrated below (Fig. 3.2).

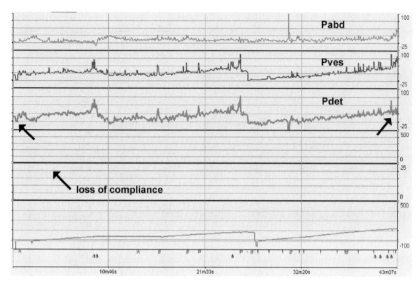

Fig. 3.2 Urodynamic trace on Oxybutinin.

1 Has Oxybutinin altered the bladder dynamics? If yes, how?
2 What alternative treatment options were available following the initial urodynamics?
3 What is the clinical management at this stage?
4 What is the likely long-term solution for this girl?

Discussion

1 It is likely that Oxybutinin has altered the bladder dynamics in this girl. The marked instability during the filling phase prior to commencement of Oxybutinin has now practically disappeared. Instead, the passive compliance of this bladder has become extremely poor. There was a rise in storage pressures of 40 cm of water for a volume instilled of 155cc. There was loss of bladder compliance from 100 ml infused, with a progressive rise in storage pressures between 100 and 155 ml infused. Toward end fill, instability was noted, with amplitude 10–15 cm of water, taking end-fill pressures up to 55 cm of water. No leakage was observed throughout the study. Oxybutinin acts by inhibiting detrusor activity, and in this patient the commencement of Oxybutinin has significantly dampened the detrusor instability. This has resulted in an increase in the dry intervals and bladder capacity. The important feature is, before commencing Oxybutinin the child was frequently wet-emptying the bladder with detrusor instability and was frequently dry afterward. Thus a safe bladder emptying by instability was suppressed by the introduction of Oxybutinin.

2 Two alternative treatment options were available following the initial urodynamic studies.

Option 1 was to offer a vesicostomy. This would allow the urine to leak freely and would decompress the lower as well as the upper urinary tract. At a later stage plans would be made to either close the vesicostomy and reassess the bladder dynamics or discuss with the family lower urinary tract reconstruction in the form of an augmentation cystoplasty with or without the creation of an ACE to deal with constipation. Bladder emptying could be achieved either through intermittent catheterization per urethra or placement of a Mitrofanoff channel.

Option 2 was to perform urethral dilatation. David Bloom et al. have showed good response to serial urethral over dilatation. Urethral dilatation reduced the incidence of urinary tract infection and has increased the bladder compliance and capacity by diminishing detrusor instability.

3 At this stage the bladder container is unsafe and stores urine at extremely high pressures, which will be detrimental to the upper urinary tract. In view of the repeat urodynamic findings, the management plan at this stage would be to create a vesicostomy and take the child off Oxybutinin.

4 The likely long-term solution for this girl would involve reconstruction of her lower urinary tract. This would involve an augmentation of her bladder using ileum and creation of an ACE to deal with constipation. As the child has been catheterized urethrally, a Mitrofanoff channel is not required, and the child would continue to catheterize and empty the augmented bladder post reconstruction via the urethral route.

Suggested reading

Austin PF, Homsy YL, Masel JL, et al. Alpha-adrenergic blockade in children with neuropathic and non-neuropathic voiding dysfunction. *J Urol.* 1999;162(3 pt 2):1064–7.

Bloom DA, Knechtel JM, McGuire EJ. Urethral dilatation improves bladder compliance in children with myelomeningocoele and high leak point pressure. *J Urol.* 1990;144(2 pt 2):430–3; discussion 443–4.

Kasabian NG, Bauer SB, Dyro FM, et al. The prophylactic value of clean intermittent catheterization and anti cholinergic medication in newborns and infants with myelodysplasia at risk of developing urinary tract deterioration. *Am J Dis Child.* 1992;146(7):840–3.

Schulte-Baukloh H, Michael T, Schobert J, et al. Efficacy of botulinum-a toxin in children with detrusor hyperreflexia due to myelomenongocoele: preliminary results. *Urology.* 2002;59(3):325–7; discussion 327–8.

Wu HY, Baskin LS, Kogan BA. Neurogenic bladder dysfunction due to myelomeningocoele: neonatal versus childhood treatment. *J Urol.* 1997;157(6):2295–7.

CASE 2

An 11-year-old boy presents with new onset of day and nighttime wetting and two symptomatic urinary tract infections over the past 3 months.

He was antenatally diagnosed to have bilateral hydronephrosis, and a postnatal diagnosis of posterior urethral valves with left vesicoureteric reflux and chronic renal failure was confirmed.

He underwent resection of the posterior urethral valves, circumcision, and a left orchidopexy. Post resection of the valves, his renal function was stable and was monitored regularly by the nephrology team.

At 5 years of age he was dry by day and mostly dry at night. A videourodynamic study demonstrated a stable compliant bladder with a capacity of 250 cc, which emptied to completion with a maximum voiding detrusor pressure of 50 cm of water and minimal left-sided reflux into the lower ureter. By the age of 7 years he was completely dry by day as well as at night. At the age of 8 years he underwent a live related renal transplant for end-stage renal failure and is currently on Cyclosporin and Azathioprine immunosuppression.

A baseline ultrasound study of his urinary tract showed the native right kidney to be small and echogenic; the left kidney was not visualized. The transplant kidney showed moderate hydronephrosis with calyceal dilatation on a full bladder. Color perfusion and spectral flow traces were normal. He voided 360 ml with postvoid residual of 50 ml. Following the void dilatation in the transplant ureter resolved leaving minimal calyceal dilatation at the upper pole.

A frequency/volume chart was obtained. It showed the first void in the morning to be 900 ml, and this was associated with a wet bed. During the day he voided 6–8 times, with a mean volume of approximately 250 cc. He was dry for the early part of the day and was damp by evening. The total input was 3 l, and the total output was 2.4 l.

Videourodynamics was performed. It showed a stable compliant bladder with a rise in pressure of 5 cm of water for 280 ml infused. The voiding phase was characterized by a maximum detrusor pressure of 29 cm of water with associated abdominal straining, resulting in a poor urinary stream. There was reflux into the transplant from 100 ml infused, and during voiding, reflux into the left native ureter was observed. He voided 295 ml, leaving a residual of approximately 30 ml (Fig. 3.3).

1 What is the likely explanation for these new symptoms?
2 What further information would be helpful in planning management?
3 What treatment options are available to alleviate the symptoms?
4 What is the natural history of the bladder in posterior urethral valves?

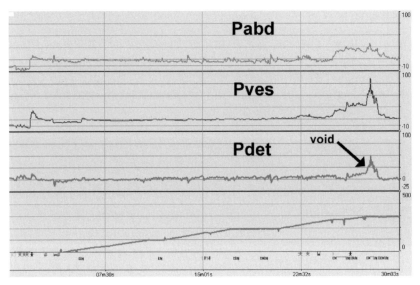

Fig. 3.3 Urodynamic trace.

Discussion

1 This is an 11-year-old boy with posterior urethral valves who was mostly dry by the age of 5 and was completely dry both by day and night by the age of 7. He has subsequently developed secondary day- and nighttime wetting.

Reviewing his 5-year urodynamic study, it was found that the voiding pressures were on the lower side of normal although he emptied his bladder to completion. Reviewing his current investigations and his frequency/volume chart, it is found that his bladder is capable of storing up to 900 cc, which is an extremely large volume for a boy of his age. Also, he tends to be dry for best part of the day and begins to get damp by evening and has a wet bed at night. This suggests that he has an overtly large capacity bladder, which does not empty to completion as shown on the ultrasound scan. The urodynamic studies confirm this suspicion as he empties the bladder with a very low rise in detrusor pressures and uses a significant amount of abdominal straining. He therefore has a decompensated bladder, and his symptoms may be exaggerated by the obligatory fluid load. Following his transplant, he has a targeted input of 3 l and therefore produces between 2.3 and 2.5 l over a 24-hour period. He has a decompensated bladder with incomplete bladder emptying and probably an overflow type of incontinence by late evening.

2 It would be useful to know his 24-hour urine output after reducing the targeted intake from 3 l to approximately 1.5 l a day. If he continues to have a large 24-hour urine output, this is most likely to be originating from his native dysplastic kidneys. If, however, reducing his targeted intake produces a significant reduction in his 24-hour urine output, then that is likely to produce an improvement in his symptomatology and may allow more efficient bladder emptying. A repeat frequency/volume chart following a period of reduced 24-hour intake would be extremely helpful in further decision making.

3 Depending on the results of his 24-hour urine production following a reduction in his targeted input, the treatment options that are available include:

a bilateral native nephrectomies if the 24-hour urine output continues to remain high following a period of fluid restriction;

b clean intermittent catheterization with continuous overnight drainage. This would ensure that the bladder is emptied to completion during the daytime and would prevent overdistension of the bladder at night. Steve Koff et al. have shown significant improvement in the bladder dynamics following introduction of this regime. It may be technically difficult for him to catheterize urethrally, and the placement of a Mitrofanoff channel may be necessary. This would facilitate catheterization during the day and would make continuous overnight drainage easier.

4 Holmdahl in 1995 in a series of papers showed the changing urodynamic pattern of the valve bladder from infancy into adolescence. In the first year of life following satisfactory valve resection, the bladders have a small capacity with detrusor instability and are hypercontractile, i.e. they have high voiding pressures. Between the age of 1 and 3 years, these bladders demonstrate an increase in capacity and reduction in the presence of hypercontractility. Holmdahl's experience with standard cystometry in boys treated for posterior urethral valves between the age of 4 and 12 years shows that the urodynamic pattern continues to change and voiding pressures continue to decrease with decrease in instability and increase in emptying difficulties.

These features are suggestive that these bladders are now decompensating. She also compared the urodynamic patterns in boys' pre- and postpuberty and found evidence of bladder decompensation in all the 6 boys who were evaluated postpuberty. These bladders had a large capacity were stable and compliant and had poor voiding detrusor pressures with large post micturition residuals. Mario DeGennaro et al. have also showed similar findings in 2000.

Suggested reading

Glassberg KI. The valve bladder syndrome: 20 years later. *J Urol.* 2001;166:1406–14.

Holmdahl G. Bladder dysfunction in boys with posterior urethral valves. *Scand J Urol Nephrol.* 1997;188(suppl):1–36.

Koff SA, Mutabagani KH, Jayanthi VR. The valve bladder syndrome: pathophysiology and treatment with nocturnal bladder emptying. *J Urol.* 2002;167(1):291–7.

Parkhouse HF, Barratt TM, Dillon MJ, et al. Long term outcome of boys with posterior urethral valves. *Br J Urol.* 1988;62:59–62.

Peters CA, Bolkier M, Bauer SB, et al. The urodynamics consequences of posterior urethral valves. *J Urol.* 1990;144:122–26.

CASE 3

A $3^1/_2$-year-old girl, with an insulin-dependent mother, presents with a history of recurrent urinary tract infections, failure to thrive, and chronic constipation.

On examination she is anemic, weighs 16 kg, and is in nappies. She has flattened buttocks and suspected sacral agenesis, and she is catheterized urethrally 5 times a day. She has not been catheterized for the last 5 days prior to presentation, and an ultrasound scan of her bladder shows a postvoid residual of a 100 cc with echogenic debris. Following a period of continuous catheter drainage and IV antibiotics, the following investigations were performed.

An ultrasound scan shows left hydroureteronephrosis, right distal dilated ureter, and a thick-walled trabeculated bladder with a postmicturition residual of 100 cc.

Baseline haematological and biochemical investigations showed:

Haemoglobin 7.5	RBC 3.91
Platelet count 581	Hct 0.250
WCC 16.2	Neutrophil 9.8
Sodium 142 (133–146)	Potassium 4.2 (3.5–5.5)
Urea 7 (2.5–6)	Creatinine 94 (20–50)
Calcium 2.29 (2.22–2.51)	Magnesium 0.9 (0.66–1)
Phosphate 1.78 (1.22–1.8)	Albumin 35 (35–52)

Urine culture grew $>10^5$ *Escherichia coli.*

DMSA scan showed multiple scars in both kidneys. Differential function was 80% for the right and 20% for the left kidney.

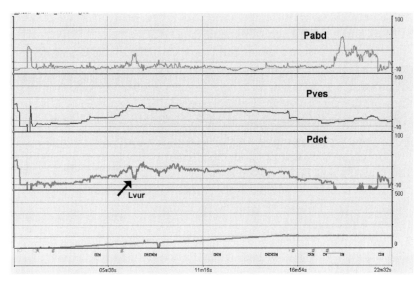

Fig. 3.4 Urodynamic trace.

Videourodynamics (Figs. 3.4 and 3.5) was performed with a 7Fg double lumen catheter per urethra, and the bladder was filled at a rate of 10–15 ml/min. Start-fill pressure was 6 cm of water, and left reflux was noted from early on during filling with approximately 40 cc infused. Gradual

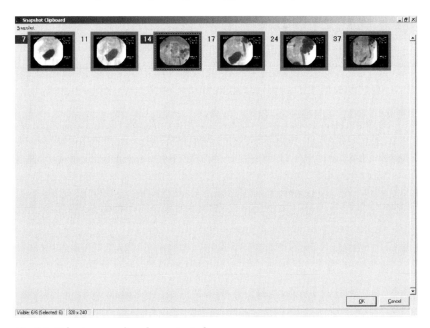

Fig. 3.5 Video images of urodynamic study.

29

rise in intravesical pressure was noted with filling, rising to 33 cm of water at 44 ml infused and 38 cm of water at 55 ml infused.

Intravesical pressure subsequently dropped with further filling, which produced distension of the left upper urinary tract. At 79 ml infused volume, the pressure was 27 cm of water and dropped to 16 cm of water at 100 ml infused. Filling was discontinued at this point, because of a gross distension of the left pelvicalyceal system and ureter. The bladder was drained of 110 ml of urine, and a further 5 ml was drained after a period of 5 minutes. Her urethral catheter was removed, and the child was recatheterized 15 minutes later and a further 80 ml was drained.

Video images showed a small trabeculated bladder with left vesicoureteric reflux grade 4/5 from approximately 40 ml infused.

1 What is the diagnosis?

2 What are the short-term and long-term treatment options?

3 How will you follow up this child?

Discussion

1 This girl has a neurogenic bladder and bowel secondary to sacral agenesis confirmed on a plain abdominal X-ray.

2 In the first instance she needs a period of continuous bladder drainage and treatment with intravenous antibiotics in order to drain the system and treat the urinary tract infection. Following a period of stabilization, one would then discuss with the family the two main options that are available in order to deal with this problem effectively.

The investigations have shown that she has an extremely small capacity bladder with very poor compliance, which generates high storage pressures.

In addition, she has gross left-sided vesicoureteric reflux into a poorly functioning kidney with bilateral renal damage secondary to the neurogenic bladder. Her renal function is significantly compromised, and she is in chronic renal failure. Even if she were to adhere to her regime of clean intermittent catheterization 4–5 times per day, she would be subjecting the upper urinary tract to prolonged periods where the storage pressures in the bladder would be extremely high.

Therefore, in the short term the safe option is to create a vesicostomy. This will allow the bladder to drain freely and will enable decompression of the upper urinary tract.

Alternatively, an elegant way of creating a diversion is a low refluxing left loop ureterostomy. The advantage of this method of decompression is that it allows the bladder to continue cycling and simultaneously prevents the high storage pressures that would potentially further damage the already compromised renal function. In general, the disadvantage of refluxing ureterostomy is that it will require closure at a later stage.

With urinary diversion in place and following a period of stabilization, the aspects of reconstructive surgery would then be discussed with the family. Reconstruction would most probably involve an augmentation ileocystoplasty and creation of an ACE. Creation of a Mitrofanoff channel is probably not required in this child because she is already accustomed to catheterizing the bladder urethrally and is the channel of choice when available. In situations where either catheterization via urethra is not possible or in female children who are wheelchair bound with neurogenic bladder or spina bifida, catheterization through the urethral route is extremely difficult and prevents self-sufficiency in this task. In these situations, consideration should be given to the placement of a Mitrofanoff channel.

The Mitrofanoff channel can be exited either into the right iliac fossa or on the left side if the patient is left handed. The cosmetic advantage of placing it into the umbilicus is an option; however, the disadvantage of an umbilical Mitrofanoff is that the catheter is directed straight at the trigone, which can occasionally cause severe discomfort and incomplete bladder emptying.

3 Following creation of vesicostomy, the child will have to be monitored with routine ultrasonography to check whether the upper tract dilatation has resolved. Renal function would be monitored closely over the following months and years to maximize the potential of the remaining functioning nephrons, and she will need nutritional supplements to overcome her growth retardation.

Following reconstructive surgery, this child will need to be followed on an annual basis. The investigations that would be performed would include routine hematological and biochemical investigations, liver and renal function assessment, and monitoring of her growth and development. A year after her reconstructive surgery, she would have a videourodynamic study, which would serve as a baseline. In the long term she will need annual check cystoscopies to monitor the bladder for development of neoplasia.

Suggested reading

Gonzalez R, Schimke CM. Strategies in urological reconstruction in myelomeningocoele. *Curr Opin Urol.* 2002;12(6):485–90.

Greenwell TJ, Venn SN, Mundy AR. Augmentation cystoplasty. *BJU Int.* 2001;88(6):511–25.

Ledermann SE, Shaw V, Trompeter RS. Long term enteral nutrition in infants and young children with chronic renal failure. *Paediatr Nephrol.* 1999;13(9):870–5.

Narayanaswamy B, Wilcox DT, Cuckow PM, et al. The Yang-Monti ileovesicostomy: a problematic channel? *BJU Int.* 2001;87(9):861–5.

Wilmhurst JM, Kelly R, Borzyskowski M. Presentation and outcome of sacral agenesis: 20 years experience. *Dev Med Child Neurol.* 1999;41(12):806–12.

CASE 4

A 27-month-old girl presents with a history of recurrent urinary tract infections requiring IV antibiotics. She was toilet trained at the age of 22 months and was dry by day but wet at night.

For the past 6 weeks she has been experiencing recurrent urinary tract infections and now has daytime frequency and urgency with incontinence in between voids. Her bowel habits are normal and physical examination is unremarkable. A baseline ultrasound scan shows two normal kidneys with an empty bladder; no dilated ureters were visualized.

In view of the recurrent urinary tract infections, she undergoes a DMSA scan and a DTPA scan with indirect cystography, which gives a differential function of 69% for the left and 31% for the right. There is scarring in the upper and lower poles of the right kidney, and on indirect cystography there is no clear evidence of vesicoureteric reflux.

A plain abdominal X-ray shows normal appearance for the bony spine and no evidence of gross constipation or calcification in the urinary tract. She had a baseline bladder function assessment, and the frequency/volume chart and flow curve are demonstrated in Figs. 3.6 and 3.7, respectively. She went on to have a suprapubic line placed in the bladder and natural fill urodynamic studies performed (Fig. 3.8). Based on the results of these investigations, an opinion was obtained from the neurosurgical team, who advised her to undergo an MRI of the spine, which was normal.

1 What is the diagnosis?

2 How will you manage this child?

3 What are the different types of nonneurogenic voiding disorders (dysfunctional voiding or dysfunctional elimination syndrome)?

Discussion

1 The diagnosis in this child is one of dysfunctional voiding. The frequency/volume chart demonstrates a series of small voids at short intervals of 30–45 minutes, the volumes ranging from 32 to 100 ml.

Date: 5.9.99

	Urine volume	(night) wet pants	Drinks volume	Drinks type	Good/bad? day/night
7:00am					
8:00am					
9:00am	woke up at 10 am		150 mls	milk	
10:00am		no pad	150 ml	milk + tea	
11:00am	1/30 30 mls, 12/0 30 mls, 12/30 100 mls	wet pants 11.30	150 ml	milk	
12 noon					
1:00pm		++	150 ml	milk	
2:00pm	75 mls				
?	20 mls	++	100 ml	coffee (no), cake	
?	75 mls	+++			
?	100 mls	++++			
?			150 ml	milk	
?		++++			Typical day
8	110 mls		150 ml milk		
9			100 mls milk		
10					
	Passed urine? happy	Wet bed?			
TLS	4389, 978 mls		1100 mls		wet very

Date: 10.9.99

	Urine volume	(day) wet pants	Drinks volume	Drinks type	Good/bad? day/night
7:00am	115 mls		150 mls	milk, bedtime	
8:00am			150 ml	-- --	
9:00am	50 ml	+			
10:00am	50 mls	+++			
11:00am	50 mls		150 ml	lemonade	
12 noon		in and out of paddling pool			quite
1:00pm	30 mls		150 ml	milk	
2:00pm	100 mls	+-			good day
3:00pm			50 ml	dilute milk	a
4:00pm	30 mls	+++			
5:00pm		++			
6:00pm			150 ml	blackcurrant	
7:00pm		asleep by 7.00pm			
8:00pm					
9:00pm					
10:00pm					
Night-time (tick)	happy	Wet bed? she was :- (!)			very dry very for Emma
TOTAL VOLUMES	549	+++	700 mls		

Fig. 3.6 Frequency/volume chart.

The flow studies on bladder function assessment show a poor flow rate with a large postmicturition residual on postvoid ultrasound.

A natural filling urodynamic study shows a stable and compliant bladder for the first 20 minutes. There is significant unstable activity on further filling, with associated urgency and minor leakages. The pressure rise with the unstable contractions is marked up to 85 cm of water, with

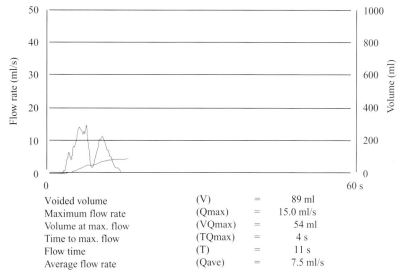

Voided volume	(V)	=	89 ml
Maximum flow rate	(Qmax)	=	15.0 ml/s
Volume at max. flow	(VQmax)	=	54 ml
Time to max. flow	(TQmax)	=	4 s
Flow time	(T)	=	11 s
Average flow rate	(Qave)	=	7.5 ml/s

Fig. 3.7 Flow curve.

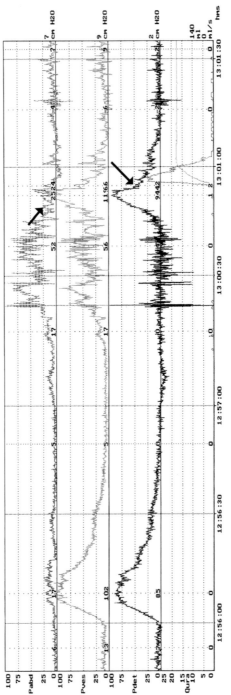

Fig. 3.8 Urodynamic trace.

an associated severe urgency to void. She voids with a maximum detrusor pressure of 94 cm of water, with increased abdominal activity before micturition and a delayed flow. The flow does not begin until the pressure drops to 35 cm of water; she then voids 140 cc with a residual of 32 cc. Therefore, combining the history and bladder function assessment along with the urodynamic study results, the diagnosis is one of dis-coordination between detrusor contraction and pelvic floor/sphincter relaxation during micturition, suggestive of dysfunctional voiding.

2 The girl was started on antibiotics; and after the acute infection had been treated, she was put on prophylactic dose of Nitrofurantoin. Simultaneously she underwent urethral dilatation, which was repeated twice with an interval of 4–6 weeks between dilatations. This resulted in a significant improvement in her urinary flow pattern; however, she continued to have significant postmicturition residuals, and therefore she was commenced on clean intermittent catheterization 4 times a day. This resulted in a significant improvement of her symptoms. Following a period of 12 months of prophylactic antibiotics and clean intermittent catheterization, she began to show a reduction in her postmicturition residuals. Antibiotic prophylaxis was stopped, and clean intermittent catheterization was reduced to twice daily.

Over the next 6 months she experienced two episodes of cystitis with dysuria and positive cultures; however, these were treated with increased fluid intake and by increasing her catheterization regime to 4 times a day. Over the last 3 months she is back to catheterization twice daily and has a more regular voiding pattern during the day. She is no longer wet in between voids and has had no further urinary tract infections.

3 This group of disorders is characterized by a completely normal physical examination, and imaging reveals no neurological abnormality. The commonest form of functional voiding disorder seen is the overactive bladder (OAB). Such children have long-standing symptoms of daytime frequency, urgency, and urge incontinence and usually have associated nocturnal enuresis.

A detailed history, frequency/volume information, flow studies with postvoid assessment of residuals, and renal ultrasound examination are used to make the diagnosis.

Urodynamic studies are indicated in protracted or resistant forms of OAB, which do not respond to conventional treatment. The majority of the studies show marked detrusor overactivity, with a reduced functional capacity and a strong associated desire to void. Sometimes, however, the urgency appears to be secondary to a precipitous drop in urethral pressure resulting in micturition (as seen on videourodynamic studies).

Vincent's courtesy is a characteristic posturing by children with OAB in an attempt to prevent wetting or voiding. The etiology of this condition is unclear and may be a result of a cerebral insult in the perinatal period, but the more commonly accepted mechanism is that these features are secondary to delayed maturation of the reticulospinal pathways and inhibitory centers in the midbrain and cerebral cortex. There may be a family history where either parent may have had similar symptoms during childhood. This suggests a genetically determined delayed rate of central nervous system maturation.

It is extremely important to investigate the bowel habit in this group of children, as occasionally children with profound constipation can develop detrusor overactivity and urinary incontinence. Similarly a child with a history of recurrent urinary tract infections may produce a similar clinical picture. In these children the detrusor overactivity occurs secondary to the inflammatory response in the bladder wall that stimulates a receptor located in the submucosa or detrusor muscle layers.

Certain foodstuffs are thought to exacerbate the symptoms, and the restriction of fizzy drinks, additives, colorants, and preservatives may improve the symptoms in the treatment of this disorder.

Ensuring a normal bowel habit and treating constipation synchronously if present is imperative in making progress in the management of these children. If urinary infection is present, it should be treated simultaneously.

Oxybutinin and more recently Tolterodine along with adequate hydration form the mainstay of treatment. More recently there have been reports of successful treatment of this condition using botulinum-A toxin. The toxin is injected endoscopically at multiple sites within the bladder in the submucosal region. It acts by blocking the muscarinic receptors within the bladder, and its action typically lasts for 6–9 months, after which it can be repeated. Its action is reversible, and systemic side effects are rare provided the recommended dosage is not exceeded.

Treatment of detrusor overactivity in boys may require a prolonged treatment over 12–24 months with Oxybutinin before a sustained response is obtained. Oxybutinin can then be tapered and discontinued.

The second and frequently more difficult functional voiding disorder to treat is the small-capacity hypertonic bladder. These children classically have a history of recurrent urinary tract infections, and the symptoms include frequency, urgency, urge incontinence, and enuresis. These symptoms persist long after the infection has been treated.

Typically, this group of children consists predominantly of girls. When the child attempts to hold back urination either because it is painful or it is inappropriate to void, they tighten or only partially relax the pelvic floor/external urinary sphincter during micturition. This produces a form of outflow obstruction disrupting the normal laminar flow pattern. This results in a stop/start staccato type of voiding pattern and may result in bacteria being milked back into the bladder, precipitating recurrent urinary tract infections.

Urodynamic studies in this group of children demonstrate a bladder with a small functional capacity when corrected for age, detrusor instability during filling, and compromised bladder compliance. At capacity there is an uncontrollable urge to void, which results in elevated detrusor voiding pressures much higher than normal values. There is dis-coordination between detrusor contraction and pelvic floor relaxation, giving rise to increased abdominal pressure resulting in incomplete bladder emptying.

In the acute stage, the management of this condition can be extremely difficult. The first line of treatment is to treat the infection, which sometimes requires IV antibiotics. This is usually followed by a period of antibiotics prophylaxis. In the older child, in addition to ensuring that all possible measures are taken as regards hygiene, the mainstay of management is to teach to try and relax completely during voiding so that a steady stream of urine is produced. This can be reinforced using biofeedback with uroflowmetry. The child should spend sufficient time on the toilet using the correct posture to ensure relaxation of the abdominal and pelvic musculature to ensure that the bladder is emptied to completion.

There have been some recent reports advocating the injection of botulinum-A toxin periurethrally. This has been reported to be successful in reversing the dis-coordination and in resistant cases allows time for biofeedback to be effective.

In the younger child these symptoms typically occur around the time of potty training, and in the more severe cases these acute symptoms can produce changes in the upper urinary tract.

Acute management may involve a period of continuous bladder drainage using either a urethral or suprapubic catheter. In addition, urethral overdilatation in combination with anticholinergic medication has been found to be useful. Institution of intermittent catheterization helps to reduce the post-micturition residuals and the risk of reinfection and is a useful adjunctive measure.

The next group of dysfunctional voiding disorder is the infrequent voider, also known as voiding postponement or lazy bladder syndrome.

This tends to affect predominantly girls who may void only once or twice during an entire 24-hour period. It is not unusual for such children to completely avoid using the toilets while at school or when they are outside the home environment. Usually these children would have had a normal voiding pattern as infants, but after potty training they have learned to withhold micturition for extended periods of time. Some children are excessively neat and may have a fetish for cleanliness that prevents them from using public bathrooms or the toilets at school.

Infrequent voiding produces a progressive increase in bladder capacity and a decrease in the stimulus to urinate. Chronically distended bladders are prone to urinary infections as well as overflow or stress incontinence. Sometimes these are the first manifestations of an abnormal voiding pattern in this group of children.

Changing the child's voiding pattern is the mainstay of treatment. Timed voiding is essential in order to retrain the bladder. Voiding every 2–3 hours by day is essential, and using a daytime alarm may be a useful adjunct to ensure compliance with the regime. These measures, along with a reassurance that it is more detrimental not to urinate than to use bathrooms that may not meet their standards of cleanliness, usually are successful in reversing the dysfunctional voiding pattern. Rarely, intermittent catheterization may be necessary for a period of time in order to allow the detrusor muscle to regain its contractile ability.

Hinman's syndrome. Children with Hinman's syndrome clinically mimic a neuropathic bladder, with no neurological abnormality that can be found on investigations. Some believe that this may be a result of persistence of the transitional phase of gaining bladder control during toilet training. Like detrusor hyperreflexia, this condition is characterized by urgency, urge incontinence, and daytime and/or nocturnal enuresis. Moreover, these children also suffer from recurrent urinary tract infections and have irregular bowel movements with fecal soiling.

Radiological investigation usually reveals profound changes within the urinary tract; hydroureteronephrosis with or without scarring is present in a large proportion of children. Approximately 50% of children have severe vesicoureteric reflux with large-capacity bladders and significant postvoid residuals. There is usually gross fecal loading consistent with chronic constipation.

There is a strong link with family dynamics, and the parents, typically the fathers, tend to be domineering and intolerant of failure. Dysfunctional families, single parents, and alcoholism are common threats that exacerbate the situation. These children are frequently punished both physically and mentally for their symptoms. Children try to withhold urination and defecation further by contracting the pelvic floor muscles, which aggravates the situation.

Urodynamic studies in this group of children typically demonstrate a large-capacity bladder, which has poor compliance with uninhibited detrusor contractions during filling. During the voiding phase, they have high pressure uncoordinated detrusor contractions with associated abdominal activity. Urinary flow is often staccato or interrupted because the pelvic floor fails to relax.

Psychotherapy forms the mainstay of treatment in this group of children. It is imperative to reeducate both the child and the parents as regards appropriate voiding habits. In a severe case, temporary urinary diversion in the form of a vesicostomy may have to be considered.

The focus of treatment is on retraining the bladder and improving the child's ability to relax the pelvic floor during voiding. Antibiotics and anticholinergic medications to inhibit detrusor instability during filling are helpful adjuncts. Despite these measures, intermittent catheterization may be required in a group of children who either fail to respond or where decompression of the upper urinary tract is of importance to prevent further damage to the kidneys.

Suggested reading

Artibani W. Diagnosis and significance of idiopathic overactive bladder. *Urology.* Dec 1997;50(6A suppl):25–32; discussion 33–5.

Cain MP, Wu SD, Austin PF, et al. Alpha-blocker therapy for children with dysfunctional voiding and urinary retention. *J Urol.* Oct 2003;170(4 pt 2):1514–15; discussion 1516–17.

Nijman RJ. Classification and treatment of functional incontinence in children. *BJU Int.* May 2000;85(suppl 3):37–42; discussion 45–6.

Pohl HG, Bauer SB, Borer JG, et al. The outcome of voiding dysfunction managed with clean intermittent catheterisation in neurologically and anatomically normal children. *BJU Int.* Jun 2002;89(9):923–7.

Schulman SL. Voiding dysfunction in children. *Urol Clin North Am.* Aug 2004;31(3):481–90.

4 | Hypospadias and Related Conditions

Warren T. Snodgrass

CASE 1

A 3-month-old male is referred for distal hypospadias.

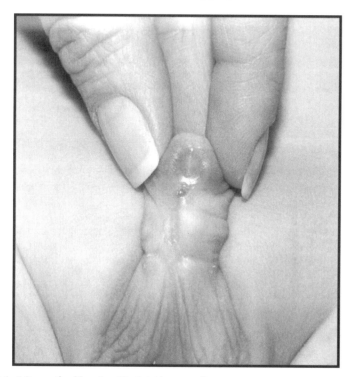

Fig. 4.1 A 3-month-old male with distal hypospadias.

1 What penile abnormalities typically occur with hypospadias?
2 How common is this condition, and what is its etiology?
3 Should additional diagnostic testing be performed to detect associated anomalies?
4 What are the indications for surgery?
5 When would you recommend correction to be performed?
6 What would you inform the parents are the expected outcomes and potential complications of surgical repair?

Discussion

1 By definition, *hypospadias* refers to a urethral meatus proximal to the usual location at the ventral tip of the glans. Extending distally from this opening is the tissue that should have tubularized to complete urethral development, referred to as the "urethral plate." In addition, most often the ventral aspect of the foreskin is deficient, resulting in a typical "hooded" appearance that calls attention to the defect during newborn examination. In approximately 15% of distal cases there will also be ventral curvature of the penis during erection that may indicate relative shortening of the ventral shaft skin, corpus spongiosum, and/or corpus cavernosa.

2 Hypospadias is considered an arrest during normal penile development that affects approximately 1 in 150–300 boys. The incidence is greater within affected families, as 7% of fathers also have hypospadias and, overall, another family member is affected in 20% of the cases. Nevertheless, most cases appear to be sporadic, and the condition has long been presumed to represent an endocrinopathy with incomplete masculinization. Chromosome abnormalities occur in less than 5% of patients with isolated hypospadias, and routine karyotyping is not recommended. Defects in testosterone production, 5-alpha-reductase II activity, and the structure and function of the androgen receptor have each been found in isolated cases. In vitro fertilization appears to result in an increased incidence of the condition, perhaps due to use of progesterones. Environmental estrogens or antiandrogens have been implicated for the reported increase in hypospadias in western societies. However, the cause for incomplete penile development remains unclear in the majority of patients.

3 The disordered embryologic events resulting in hypospadias occur following the eighth week of gestation, after the ureteral bud induces renal development. Therefore, upper tract imaging is not necessary, and in most boys hypospadias occurs as an isolated anomaly.

4 There are both functional and cosmetic reasons to consider surgical correction for distal hypospadias. The proximal location of the meatus may result in a broad, deflected urinary stream that will be difficult to reliably direct after toilet training when the boy stands to void. Furthermore, the hooded prepuce is visibly abnormal and may be a source of ridicule from others. While most boys with distal hypospadias either have no, or only mild, ventral curvature with erection, an occasional patient has sufficient bending to impact sexual functioning as an adult.

5 The normal postnatal surge in testosterone results in phallic growth sufficient to consider outpatient hypospadias repair as early as 3 months of age in otherwise healthy boys. In former premature infants, surgery is delayed

for anesthetic considerations until at least 6 months. Because of increasing awareness of the genitalia with age, it is considered best to complete surgery whenever possible before children reach 2 years of age.

6 Following description of the MAGPI procedure in 1981, interest in distal hypospadias surgery increased as operations to correct the defect became more reliable with fewer complications. There are a variety of techniques in current use for distal hypospadias, but all these are intended to reposition the meatus at the normal tip of the glans. The abnormal foreskin can be reconstructed to correct the ventral deficiency and give the appearance that the penis was never operated, or it can be removed for circumcision (Fig. 4.2). The most common complication from urethroplasty is fistulas, followed by meatal stenosis or neourethral stricture and wound dehiscence. The expected rate of complications is approximately 5% in currently used distal repairs.

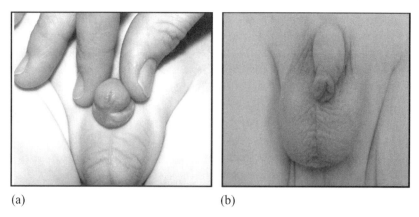

(a)   (b)

Fig. 4.2 Postoperative result after hypospadias repair (a) with circumcision and (b) with foreskin reconstructed.

Suggested reading

Bauer SB, Retik AB, Colodny AH. Genetic aspects of hypospadias. *Urol Clin North Am.* 1981;8:559–64.

Erdenetsetseg G, Dewan PA. Reconstruction of the hypospadiac hooded prepuce. *J Urol.* 2003;169:1822–24.

Moreno-Garcia M, Miranda EB. Chromosomal anomalies in cryptorchidism and hypospadias. *J Urol.* 2002;168:2170–72.

Thomas DFM. Hypospadiology: science and surgery. *BJU Int.* 2004;93:470–73.

Snodgrass W. Tubularized incised plate repair for distal hypospadias. *Atlas Urol Clin.* 2003;11:1–6.

CASE 2

This infant is referred with proximal hypospadias.

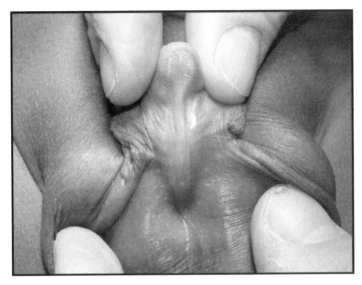

Fig. 4.3 Infant with proximal hypospadias.

1 Should further evaluation and therapy be considered before undertaking surgical correction?
2 What is the likelihood that a child with proximal hypospadias will still have ventral curvature after the penis is degloved, and what are the options to consider for its correction?
3 Describe in general terms techniques for urethroplasty in this patient.
4 What are the complication rates from proximal hypospadias repair?

Discussion

1 Although the extent of the penile anomaly is obviously greater with proximal than distal hypospadias, there should be no increased risk for upper urinary tract problems as already discussed above. However, approximately 10% of boys with penoscrotal to perineal hypospadias will have an enlarged prostatic utricle that may cause difficulty with urethral catheterization. The phallus may also be smaller in more severe cases of hypospadias, and curvature sometimes complicates preoperative assessment of penile size. It is easier to evaluate size of the glans, and androgen stimulation is recommended when it appears small. Testosterone cream or injections of either testosterone or hCG have been used, but the parenteral route is considered more reliable. Perhaps most commonly, 2 or 3 injections of testosterone enanthate 2 mg/kg are given intramuscularly at intervals of 3– 4 weeks before surgery.

2 Over 50% of boys with proximal hypospadias have ventral penile curvature after the shaft skin is released. Traditionally this bending was referred to as "chordee" and thought to result from dysgenic dartos fascia, Buck's fascia, and corpus spongiosum on the ventral shaft. Straightening involved excision of these tissues, including those now recognized as the urethral plate. Realization that bending often persisted despite even extensive dissection along the ventral shaft, coupled with interest in preserving the urethral plate for urethroplasty, has influenced methods used for correcting "chordee." Today mild curvature usually is straightened by 1 or 2 dorsal midline plication stitches. Mobilization of the corpus spongiosum adjacent to the urethral plate off the underlying corpora cavernosa can decrease or resolve bending, and this dissection can be continued under the entire plate if curvature persists. When these maneuvers are not sufficient, the urethral plate is transected. This maneuver sometimes corrects bending, or it reduces its extent so that dorsal plication can be performed. Persistent, severe curvature should be corrected by ventral corporal grafting to lengthen the shortened aspect of the corpora cavernosa.

3 The challenge in hypospadias urethroplasty is to construct a tube from the meatus to the tip of the glans. This can be accomplished by tubularization of the urethral plate or through use of various flaps or grafts. Furthermore, surgery can be done in either 1 or 2 stages. When curvature is resolved with preservation of the urethral plate and the plate is supple, tubularized incised plate urethroplasty is an increasingly popular option, although onlay prepucial flaps are also commonly used in this circumstance. If the plate is transected for straightening, tubularized prepucial flaps are preferred by some as a one-stage procedure, whereas others instead rely upon a two-step repair, transposing prepucial skin to the ventral shaft at the first operation for subsequent tubularization at the second. Grafts from skin, bladder mucosa, or buccal mucosa have also been used as onlay patches or tubes, although less commonly in primary surgery than in reoperations.

4 Complications occur more often following proximal hypospadias surgery than with distal repairs. Rates ranging from as low as 5% to over 50% have been reported for the various techniques mentioned above. Meticulous attention to technical details reduces problems, and some general principles can be applied to different surgical procedures. To avoid fistulas,

epithelium of the neourethra should be turned into the lumen with subepithelial stitches, and barrier layers placed between the urethral and overlying skin closures. The segments of corpus spongiosum running alongside the urethral plate can be mobilized sufficiently to realign them in the midline over the neourethra (the so-called "Y to I" maneuver), and then a pedicle of dartos obtained from the prepuce and dorsal shaft skin can additionally be used to give two-layer coverage. Similarly, the vascular pedicle to prepucial flaps should be advanced over the neourethral suture line. Diverticula are very unusual after urethral plate tubularization, but do occur with both onlay and tubularized prepucial flaps. Care should be taken to avoid oversizing these flaps, but diverticulum formation can still occur – presumably from the distensability of prepucial skin and the irregular lumen flaps created within the neourethra. Meatal stenosis can result from overzealous closure of the distal aspect of the neourethra or postoperative scarring. Strictures are considered a problem with the circular anastomosis of tubularized flaps to the native meatus, which accordingly should be widely spatulated. Onlay flaps and urethral plate tubularization have a lower incidence of strictures than tubularized flaps.

There is no clear advantage among various suture materials available for repair, and 6-0 and 7-0 absorbable sutures generally are preferred in infants and young boys. The likelihood that suture tracks will form may be diminished by subepithelial skin closure. Urinary diversion is provided by 6FR or 8FR stents dripping into diapers for at least one week. An antibiotic such as trimethoprim-sulfamethoxazole is prescribed postoperatively while the stent is in place.

Suggested reading

Cheng EY, Vemulapalli SN, Kropp BP, Pope JC IV, Furness PD III, Kaplan WE, Smith DP. Snodgrass hypospadias repair with vascularized dartos flap: the perfect repair for virgin cases of hypospadias? *J Urol.* 2002;168:1723–36.

FeFoor W, Wacksman J. Results of single staged hypospadias surgery to repair penoscrotal hypospadias with bifid scrotum or penoscrotal transposition. *J Urol.* 2003;170: 1585–8.

Greenfield S, Sadler B, Wan J. Two-stage repair for severe hypospadias. *J Urol.* 1994;152: 498–501.

Snodgrass W, Mitchell ME. New concepts regarding chordee and the urethral plate in hypospadias surgery. *AUA Update Ser.* 1999;28:210–15.

Yerkes E, Adams M, Miller DA, Pope JC IV, Rink RC, Brock JW III. Y to I wrap: use of distal spongiosum for hypospadias repair. *J Urol.* 2000;163:1536–9.

CASE 3

This child has persistent hypospadias despite several attempts at repair.

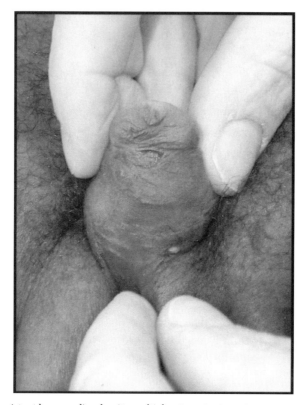

Fig. 4.4 Persistent hypospadias despite multiple attempts at repair.

1 What preoperative assessments and therapy should be considered?
2 What surgical techniques currently are recommended for hypospadias re-operations?

Discussion

1 The history should review prior operations and current symptoms, including curvature with erection, leakage from fistulas, a slow stream suggesting stenosis or stricture, and/or ballooning of the urethra from a diverticulum. Physical examination evaluates the meatal location, status of the urethral plate, availability of genital skin, hair within the urethra, and unsightly scars or irregular shaft skin. Testosterone therapy may be considered in prepubertal boys to possibly improve vascularity to penile

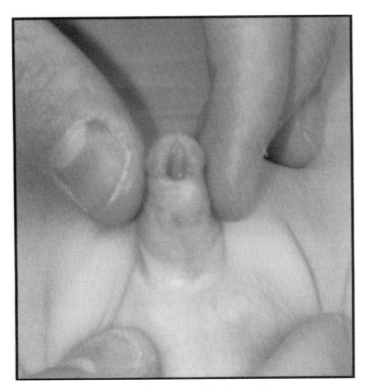

Fig. 4.7 Abnormal-appearing glanular meatus after circumcision.

1 What is the diagnosis? Is this an injury from circumcision?
2 How does this anomaly differ from "typical" distal hypospadias?
3 How is this problem corrected?

Discussion

1 This patient has the so-called megameatus intact prepuce (MIP) variant of distal hypospadias. It is important to recognize that this is not the result of a "botched" circumcision. These boys have a normal-appearing penis, and so the defect is not encountered until the foreskin becomes retractable or circumcision is performed.

2 There are several differences between MIP and typical distal hypospadias. Obviously, MIP by definition is associated with a completely formed prepuce in contrast to the ventrally deficient foreskin in other cases of hypospadias. Furthermore, the meatus is abundantly large in the MIP variant, whereas many boys with distal hypospadias have a rather small-appearing meatus. Ventral curvature is much less likely to occur in a patient with MIP than in those with other varieties of distal hypospadias.

3 Correction basically involves tubularization of the urethral plate to move the meatus to the glans tip. Because the urethral plate is larger than usual in these boys, a relaxing incision is not generally needed as with TIP repair, although when the plate is flat, incision will help "hinge" it to create a vertical and slit meatus. Some patients have a transverse web of skin distal to the meatus, and this should be excised to prevent deflection of the urinary stream. Care must be exercised when separating the glans wings from the urethral plate, since the plate in MIP patients sometimes extends more laterally than is usual in routine distal hypospadias patients. The author uses a Y-shaped incision when prior circumcision has been done; the lateral incisions along the margins of the urethral plate and glans wings joining in the midline proximal to the meatus and then extending toward the penoscrotal junction. The plate is tubularized and then a dartos pedicle flap is created from the ventral surface to cover the neourethra. Glansplasty is performed, and excess ventral shaft skin is excised as needed to optimize the cosmetic appearance.

Suggested reading

Duckett JW, Keating MA. Technical challenge of the megameatus intact prepuce hypospadias variant. *J Urol.* 1989;141:1407–9.

Hill GA, Wacksman J, Lewis AG, Sheldon CA. The modified pyramid hypospadias procedure: repair of megameatus and deep glanular groove variants. *J Urol.* 1993;150:1208–11.

CASE 6

This boy is noted to have hypospadias and a nonpalpable testis on one side. He is otherwise thought to be healthy, and there is no family history known to his mother for either anomaly.

1 Describe additional evaluation to consider in this child.

2 What are the most likely findings?

3 How commonly are intersex conditions encountered in boys with both an undescended testis and hypospadias?

Discussion

1 The finding of both cryptorchidism and hypospadias should prompt consideration of an underlying intersex disorder. Therefore it is reasonable in

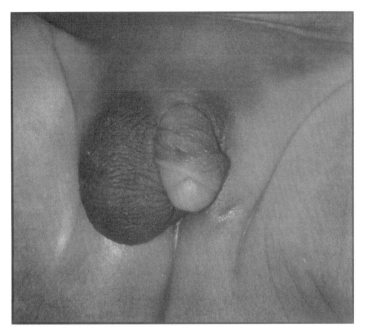

Fig. 4.8 Hypospadias and a nonpalpable testis on one side.

this case to obtain a karyotype before proceeding with surgical intervention.

2 Most often a karyotype obtained because of cryptorchidism and hypospadias will be normal, indicating no intersex condition. The most common abnormality found is mixed gonadal dysgenesis with a 45X0/46XY mosaicism. The nonpalpable testis in this situation is a streak, and Müllerian structures, including a fallopian tube, rudimentary uterus, and vagina, are additionally found since the streak does not produce Müllerian inhibiting substance. True hermaphrodites can also present with the combination of undescended testis and hypospadias. In the newborn period the finding of bilaterally nonpalpable testes and hypospadias should raise concerns for female pseudohermaphroditism associated with congenital adrenal hyperplasia. In one sense both cryptorchidism and hypospadias could be considered evidence of incomplete masculinization within the spectrum of male pseudohermaphroditism, but in the absence of a defined condition these are not included as intersex problems.

3 The incidence of intersexuality when both cryptorchidism and hypospadias occur has been reported in 25% to 33% of patients. The likelihood increases if the undescended testis is not palpable, and similarly it is greater as the severity of the hypospadias defect increases. However, in reported

series, not all patients have undergone karyotyping; so the incidence of intersexuality may have been underestimated, especially when the undescended testis could be palpated and the meatus was on the distal shaft or glans. Furthermore, when the karyotype is 46XY and the penis is not significantly diminished in size, endocrine testing has not been done routinely to detect various conditions comprising male pseudohermaphroditism.

Suggested reading

Kaefer M, Diamond D, Hendren WH, et al. The incidence of intersexuality in children with cryptorchidism and hypospadias: stratification based on gonadal palpability and meatal position. *J Urol.* 1999;162:1003–1006.

McAleer IM, Kaplan GW. Is routine karyotyping necessary in the evaluation of hypospadias and cryptorchidism? *J Urol.* 2001;165:2029–31.

5 | Testicular Disorders

John M. Park and Peter C. Fisher

CASE 1

An 11-month-old boy is referred for evaluation of a missing left testicle. According to the parents and the pediatrician, the left testicle has never been palpable in the scrotum since birth. The child has been healthy otherwise. On physical examination, the right testicle is easily found in the scrotal sac and is palpably normal, along with normally distinguishable epididymis and spermatic cord. The left testicle can be palpated using bimanual examination in the inguinal region but cannot be brought down to the scrotum.

1 What are the management options and their rationale?
2 What is the most reliable way to locate a missing testicle?
3 How should a nonpalpable testicle be managed?
4 What are the prognostic implications for patients with cryptorchidism?

Discussion

1 The first main objective in the evaluation of patients with cryptorchidism (hidden or missing testicle) is to distinguish whether the situation represents a true ectopic undescended testicle, or a retractile testicle. A retractile testicle is caused by hyperactive cremasteric muscle contraction, which temporarily pulls the testicle into the inguinal region, but the testicle can be easily brought down to the bottom of the scrotum using gentle bimanual technique (Fig. 5.1). Once brought down, a retractile testicle should be associated with minimal upward tension on the spermatic cord. In most situations, a retractile testicle is not a surgical problem and may be followed with periodic examinations. In the case of a true ectopic undescended testicle, the recommended management is watchful waiting during the first 6 months of life, and surgical orchidopexy if it persists beyond 6 months of age. Some advocate the use of human chorionic gonadotropin (hCG) to stimulate testicular descent. The success rate of hCG stimulation is variable and may be more effective for lower undescended testicles (e.g. lying at external inguinal ring or beyond). It may also aid in distinguishing true ectopic testicles from retractile testicles. Operative orchidopexy is highly successful and remains the gold standard. The indications for

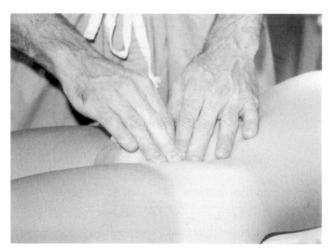

Fig. 5.1 Cryptorchidism: bimanual examination technique.

intervention include optimal testicular development and maturation for spermatogenesis and a more effective postpubertal tumor surveillance.

2 Scrotal sonography can detect testicles within the inguinal region but is limited in distinguishing retractile versus undescended testicles. Computed tomography (CT) and magnetic resonance imaging (MRI) are much more sensitive in terms of localization, especially for detecting intra-abdominal testicles. In managing inguinal testicles, however, imaging studies rarely provide any additional information to that obtained by a careful physical examination in preoperative planning. Imaging studies are neither sensitive nor specific enough to obviate the need for surgical exploration in patients with a missing testicle.

3 When a testicle is not palpable, it may represent either an intra-abdominal testicle or a vanishing testicle syndrome (testicular agenesis). Although CT and MRI can aid in localization, diagnostic laparoscopy remains the gold standard in formulating therapeutic plan. Laparoscopy not only establishes the presence of intra-abdominal testicle but also provides immediate information regarding the quality and location of the testicle for surgical intervention. If the laparoscopy indicates an intra-abdominal testicle of good quality (Fig. 5.2), it may be brought down by either one-step or two-step (following the staged Fowler–Stephens principle) orchidopexy. If the laparoscopy indicates blind-ending gonadal vessels and vas deferens, in conjunction with a nonpalpable testicle on physical examination, then the child is declared to have a vanishing testicle syndrome, and a further search for the ipsilateral testicular tissue becomes unnecessary. If the laparoscopy indicates viable gonadal vessels and vas deferens exiting

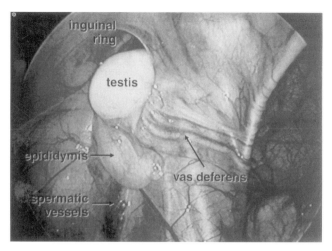

Fig. 5.2 Cryptorchidism: laparoscopic view of intra-abdominal testicle.

through the internal inguinal ring, an inguinal and/or scrotal exploration must be performed to confirm the presence or absence of viable testicular tissue. When both testicles are not palpable, one must raise a suspicion for possible intersex conditions, and karyotype and hormonal profile should be characterized. The serum level of Müllerian inhibiting substance (MIS) is extremely specific and sensitive in determining the presence or absence of functional testicular tissue in patients with bilateral cryptorchidism. An hCG stimulation test will also reveal the presence of testicular tissue if an appropriate testosterone surge is noted.

4 Parents and patients should be counseled that boys with undescended testicles may have diminished fertility potential in the future. Available evidence suggests that boys with unilateral undescended testicles have a better fertility outcome than those with either bilateral undescended or intra-abdominal testicles. The benefit of early orchidopexy is debated but not proven. Undescended testicles also exhibit increased potential for germ cell malignancy postpubertally, most commonly seminoma. Surgical orchidopexy may not decrease the actual biological risk of testicular cancer, but a scrotal location provides a great advantage by allowing regular self-examination and early detection. Parents and patients should be instructed to perform biweekly testicular self-examinations after the onset of puberty.

Suggested reading

Barthold JS, Gonzalez R. The epidemiology of congenital cryptorchidism, testicular ascent and orchidopexy. *J Urol.* 2003;170(6):2396–401.

Miller OF, Stock JA, Cilento BG, McAleer IM, Kaplan GW. Prospective evaluation of human chorionic gonadotropin in the differentiation of undescended testes from retractile testes. *J Urol.* 2003;169(6):2328–31.

Rozanski T, Bloom D. The undescended testis: theory and management. *Urol Clin North Am.* 1995;22(1):107–118.

CASE 2

A 2-year-old boy presents with right scrotal swelling. It was first noted by his parents during bathing 1 month ago. He reports no pain and is voiding without difficulty. Examination reveals normal external genitalia with enlarged right hemiscrotum. The enlarged scrotum transmits light easily (positive transillumination) (Fig. 5.3), and the scrotum is neither tense nor tender. The testicle and epididymis are not easily palpable due to the scrotal swelling. The spermatic cord above the scrotum feels moderately thickened. The left scrotum and contents are normal.

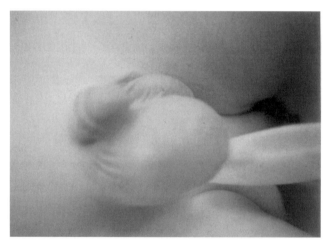

Fig. 5.3 Hydrocele: scrotal transillumination.

1 What are the possible etiologies for this presentation?
2 What are the key aspects of evaluation?
3 What are the treatment options?
4 What are the indication and rationale for exploring the normal contralateral scrotum?

Discussion

1 Painless scrotal enlargement can be caused by invaginating tissues from the inguinal region such as hernia or communicating hydrocele. A noncommunicating hydrocele can occur rarely in toddlers after trauma or epididymo-orchitis. Other possible diagnostic entities include varicocele (rare in prepubertal boys), neoplasm, lymphedema, and testicular hypertrophy. Rarely, infectious, inflammatory, and ischemic conditions such as epididymo-orchitis and spermatic cord torsion can present with minimal symptoms, but they are unlikely to persist after 1 month without clinical progression.

2 An ability to palpate and distinguish intrascrotal contents is critical to differentiate testicular parenchymal problems from paratesticular ones. Scrotal contents that transilluminate favor a fluid-filled enlargement such as hydrocele. Palpating a thickened spermatic cord and reducing the size of fluid collection manually suggest a communicating hydrocele with patent processus vaginalis. Scrotal sonography is recommended for a tense hydrocele and in postpubertal males to ensure the integrity of the testicle.

3 In infants with nontense hydrocele, observation is recommended initially, and in most cases it will resolve spontaneously. Surgery should be considered for a very tense and large hydrocele, as well as a progressively enlarging hydrocele. During observation, the parents should be instructed regarding possible risk of intra-abdominal content herniation and incarceration such as omentum and bowel. The hydrocele should be approached through an inguinal incision in order to decompress the hydrocele sac and to high-ligate the patent processus vaginalis at the internal inguinal ring.

4 When and how to explore the contralateral inguinal canal for subclinical inguinal hernia or communicating hydrocele remains debatable. One can perform a quick diagnostic laparoscopic inspection of the contralateral internal inguinal ring through the hernia sac (the process is called hernioscopy). Some advocate routine contralateral exploration in infants younger than 2 years because of high incidence of subclinical hernia.

Suggested reading

Lym L, Ross JH, Alexander F, Kay R. Risk of contralateral hydrocele or hernia after unilateral hydrocele repair in children. *J Urol.* 1999;169:1169–70.

Schneck FX, Bellinger MF. Abnormalities of the testes and scrotum and their surgical management. In: Walsh PC, Retik AB, Vaughan ED, Wein AJ, eds. *Campbell's Urology.* 8th ed. Philadelphia: Saunders; 2002.

Skoog SJ, Conlin MJ. Pediatric hernias and hydroceles: the urologist's perspective. *Urol Clin North Am.* 1995;22:119–30.

Yerkes EB, Brock JW III, Holcomb GW III, Morgan WM III. Laparoscopic evaluation for a contralateral patent processus vaginalis: part III. *Urology.* 1998;51:480–83.

CASE 3

A 10-year-old boy presents for evaluation of dull right-sided testicular pain lasting several weeks. There is no history of scrotal trauma or infection. Urinalysis is normal, and physical examination reveals normal intrascrotal contents, including normal, symmetrical testicles bilaterally. Scrotal sonography shows multiple hyperechoic foci of 1–2 mm in diameter, randomly distributed through both testicles. No other testicular parenchymal abnormality is seen, and the surrounding peritesticular structures are all normal (Fig. 5.4).

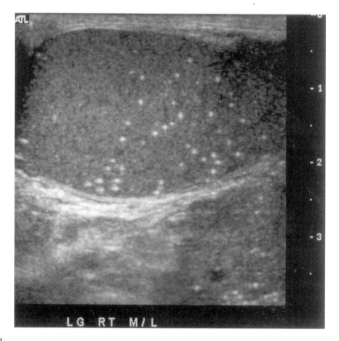

Fig. 5.4

1 What is the diagnosis?
2 What are some of the associated conditions?
3 What is the reasonable evaluation and management of this condition?
4 When is testicular biopsy indicated?

Discussion

1 The sonographic findings are consistent with testicular microlithiasis. Testicular microlithiasis is usually an incidental finding in male patients between adolescence and 50 years of age. The true incidence of testicular

microlithiasis in prepubertal boys is unknown, but some have reported finding testicular microlithiasis from <1% to 6.7% in pediatric autopsy specimens. In rare cases, patients with testicular microlithiasis present with nonspecific chronic orchalgia, but in most cases it is asymptomatic.

2 Testicular microlithiasis has been seen in patients with various testicular pathologies, such as testicular malignancy, subfertility, cryptorchidism, varicocele, testicular torsion, and testicular trauma, and in other syndromes where systemic microcalcifications are found.

3 Careful history and physical examination along with serum tumor markers (alpha-fetoprotein and beta-human chorionic gonadotropin) should be obtained during the initial evaluation. Older boys should be educated to perform a proper testicular self-examination regularly and reminded of the increased risk of testicular malignancy. The exact incidence of malignancy is not established, but the strongest evidence for this speculation comes from the higher observed rate of testicular microlithiasis in patients with known germ cell malignancy. Therefore, patients are recommended for annual physical examination, serum tumor markers, and scrotal sonography until they are beyond the risk age for germ cell malignancy. Orchalgia associated with testicular microlithiasis may be treated with nonsteroidal anti-inflammatory drugs.

4 Concerns regarding possible malignancy are the primary indication for testicular biopsy in patients with testicular microlithiasis. Those presenting with either a focal or unilateral testicular microlithiasis should be considered for biopsy – especially patients with prior history of cryptorchidism and germ cell malignancy.

Suggested reading

Furness PD, Hann LE, Hadar O, et al. Testicular microlithiasis: what is its association with testicular cancer? *Radiology.* 2001;220(1):70–75.

Hobarth K, Susani M, Szabo N. Incidence of testicular microlithiasis. *Urology.* 1992;40:464–7.

Miller RL, Wissman R, White S, et al. Testicular microlithiasis: a benign condition with a malignant association. *J Clin Ultrasound.* 1996;24:197–202.

Rosenfield AT. Proper management of a patient with testicular microlithiasis but not tumor on sonography. *AJR.* 1994;163(4):988–99.

CASE 4

A 13-year-old boy presents for evaluation of painless left scrotal mass detected on self-examination. He denies any history of scrotal trauma or infection. He has no voiding difficulties. The mass is round and compressible, measuring approximately 1 cm in diameter at the upper pole region of the epididymis, and is clearly separate from the testicle. It also transilluminates easily. The rest of the physical examination is normal. Scrotal sonography reveals a round, fluid-filled mass near the epididymis, which is clearly separate from the normal-appearing testicle (Fig. 5.5).

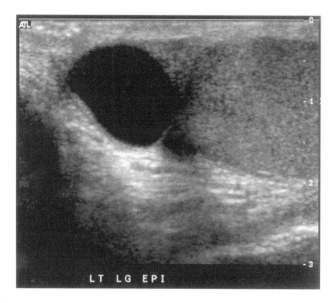

Fig. 5.5

1 What is the most likely diagnosis?
2 What are other differential diagnostic possibilities?
3 What are the typical diagnostic criteria?
4 What are the treatment options?

Discussion

1 Epididymal cyst (also called spermatocele) is the most common paratesticular mass. Epididymal cyst is usually seen near the head of the epididymis and is typically asymptomatic. Epididymal cyst forms as a result of epididymal tubule obstruction, resulting in spermatozoa-filled cyst (hence the synonym spermatocele). Tubule obstruction typically occurs in the rete testis or the epididymis and may develop after scrotal trauma or epididymo-orchitis. Patients with von Hipple–Lindau disease have an increased frequency of epididymal cysts, and approximately 20% of male

offspring of women treated with diethylstilbesterol during pregnancy may also develop epididymal cysts.

2 Other fluid-filled scrotal masses include hydrocele and varicocele, which are easily distinguished on the basis of physical examination and imaging studies. Solid paratesticular masses in this age group include benign entities (most commonly adenomatoid tumor) and malignant rhabdomyosarcoma.

3 Important diagnostic features of the physical examination include a compressible mass that is clearly separate from the testicle and transilluminates easily. A firm mass that is contiguous with the testicle should be evaluated aggressively as a possible germ cell malignancy. Lack of transillumination suggests a solid mass rather than a fluid-filled one and may represent a malignant tumor. Sonography is both sensitive and specific to address both of these concerns accurately.

4 Epididymal cysts are usually asymptomatic and require no treatment. When painful, a short course treatment with nonsteroidal anti-inflammatory drugs may be employed. Percutaneous sclerotherapy has been tried but with a high recurrence rate. Scrotal exploration with epididymal cyst excision is curative in the case of large or symptomatic cysts. Typically, epididymal cysts have no significant impact on fertility. There have been few case reports in which massively enlarged cysts have caused epididymal obstruction.

Suggested reading

Hermans BP, Foster RS, Donohue JP. Paratesticular masses. *AUA Update Ser.* 1998; 17(37):289–96.

Schneck FX, Bellinger MF. Abnormalities of the testes and scrotum and their surgical management. In: Walsh PC, Retik AB, Vaughan ED, Wein AJ, eds. *Campbell's Urology.* 8th ed. Philadelphia: Saunders; 2002.

Vohra S, Morgentaler A. Congenital anomalies of the vas deferens, epididymis, and seminal vesicles. *Urology.* 1997;49(3):313–21.

CASE 5

A 4-year-old boy presents with a painful, swollen scrotum. The symptoms began 6 hours ago, when he woke up from sleep because of pain. The patient has vomited twice since the onset of pain but has not noted any fever or voiding difficulties. On examination, his left hemiscrotum is enlarged, firm, and tender to palpation (Fig. 5.6). The left testicle cannot be distinguished from the epididymis due to swelling and tenderness. Cremasteric reflex is absent on the left side. The right testicle, epididymis, and spermatic cord are normal. Urinalysis is unremarkable.

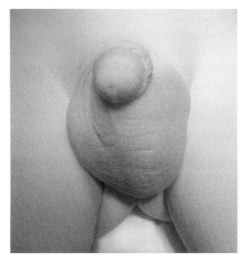

Fig. 5.6 Acute scrotum: enlarged scrotum.

1 What is the differential diagnosis?
2 How should this be evaluated?
3 What is the indication for surgical exploration?
4 How does this presentation differ from that of a newborn?

Discussion

1 The possible causes of an acute scrotum include spermatic cord torsion, inflamed hydrocele, incarcerated hernia, genital trauma, infectious epididymo-orchitis, and neoplasia. Occasionally, idiopathic scrotal edema can present with acute scrotal swelling. In this case presentation, spermatic cord torsion is the most likely diagnosis, in that (i) its onset was sudden, (ii) it was associated with other systemic symptoms such as emesis, (iii) cremasteric reflex was absent and there was high-riding testicle on examination, and (iv) urinalysis was normal.

2 Spermatic cord torsion is a urologic emergency and a prompt detorsion must be accomplished to restore testicular blood flow. If the index of suspicion is high, as was in this case, one must not delay detorsion because of diagnostic maneuvers. In uncertain situations, one can rely on Doppler scrotal sonography and nuclear testicular scan to assess blood flow. Rarely, detorsion can be achieved without surgical exploration, and this approach

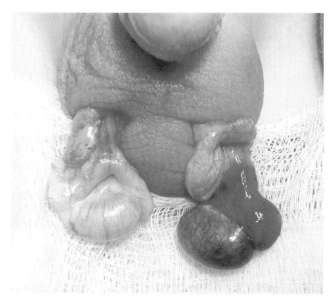

Fig. 5.7 Acute scrotum: surgical exploration of spermatic cord torsion.

may require parenteral sedation and analgesia. The danger with nonoperative detorsion is that one cannot be certain of the direction of torsion and may make the situation worse.

3 Salvage rate of the testicle after spermatic cord torsion is inversely proportional to the ischemia time; therefore, prompt evaluation and intervention are critical. Testicular salvage rate drops off significantly beyond 6 hours of complete ischemia (Fig. 5.7). Even if the involved testicle is not thought to be salvageable due to late presentation, one must not delay the intervention, since the spermatic cord may twist intermittently and the testicle may still be viable. Furthermore, the anatomic defect of horizontal lie and a "bell-clapper" deformity may exist in the contralateral testicle, which should be surgically repaired to prevent torsion.

4 Spermatic cord torsion in the newborns differs from that of older children and adolescents. In the newborns, spermatic cord torsion occurs outside the tunica vaginalis because of abnormality in the gubernacular attachment. In contrast, in the older children and adolescents, spermatic cord torsion occurs within the tunica vaginalis because of abnormal posterior attachment and horizontal lie (bell-clapper deformity). Salvage rate for newborn torsion is extremely low. Perinatal torsion is thought to occur either during or before delivery. Furthermore, surveillance of torsion symptoms is extremely difficult in newborns. As in adolescents, the anatomic abnormality of abnormal gubernacular fixation likely exists on the contralateral side; therefore, a prompt scrotal exploration and orchidopexy is recommended.

Suggested reading

Jefferson RH, Perez LM, Joseph DB. Critical analysis of the clinical presentation of acute scrotum: a 9-year experience at a single institution. *J Urol*. 1997;158(3):1198–200.

Kadish HA, Bolte RG. A retrospective review of pediatric patients with epididymitis, testicular torsion, and torsion of the testicular appendages. *Pediatrics*. 1998;102(1):73–6.

Noske HD, Kraus SW, Altinkilic BM, Weidner W. Historical milestones regarding torsion of the scrotal organs. *J Urol*. 1998;159(1):13–16.

Rabinowitz R, Hulbert WC. Acute scrotal swelling. *Urol Clin North Am*. 1995;22(1):155.

6 | Epispadias, Bladder and Cloacal Exstrophy

John P. Gearhart

CASE 1

Three patients are shown in Fig. 6.1 (a,b,c).

1 How would you describe patient A, patient B, and patient C?
2 What is the incidence and sex ratio in bladder exstrophy?
3 Are there pelvic anomalies associated with these defects?
4 Are there pelvic soft tissue defects associated with this defect?
5 What would you tell the family about the timing of surgery and eventual continence?
6 What would you tell them about sexual function and eventual fertility?

Discussion

1 *Patient A* is a male with classic bladder exstrophy. The lower urinary tract is open from the dome of the bladder to the tip of the penis. The patient has a very good sized bladder template and a good-sized penis and urethral groove.

   Patient B has a reasonable phallus for a newborn exstrophy but a small inelastic bladder template covered with hamartomatous polyps unsuitable for repair.

   Patient C is a female with a good-sized bladder template, a bifid clitoris, and a wide-open urethral plate and is open from the dome of the bladder to the tip of the urethra. The labia minora are small and the vaginal opening lies between them.

2 The incidence of bladder exstrophy is 1 in 30,000–50,000 live births. The sex ratio is 5:1 male to female.

3 Pelvic anomalies associated with bladder exstrophy include a 30% shortage of bone in the pubis, 18° external rotation of the anterior pelvis, and 14° anterior rotation of the posterior pelvis. There is also a 10–11° external rotation of the sacroiliac joint and a 15° superior/inferior rotation of the pelvis.

4 The soft tissue defects associated with bladder exstrophy include a levator hiatus that is 1.3 times wider and 2 times longer than normal.

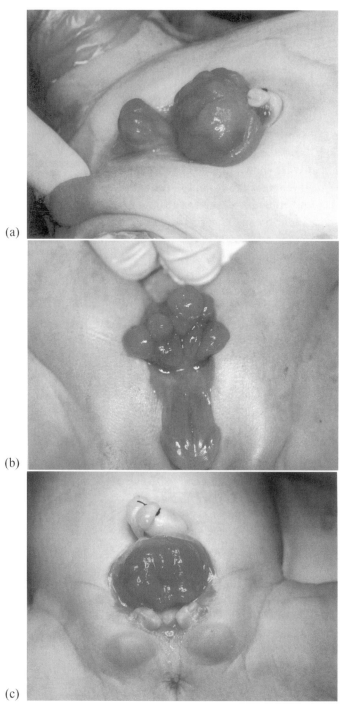

Fig. 6.1

Seventy percent of the levator ani muscle complex is located behind the rectum and only 30% anterior to the rectum supporting the anterior pelvic structures.

5 You should counsel the family that in the male, closure of the bladder with closure of the posterior urethra should occur in the first 48 hours of life. In the female the bladder, urethra, and external genitalia are all repaired in the newborn period. In *select* newborns, delayed primary closures and reclosures and the bladder and epispadias repair are done concomitantly. This is to take advantage of the maternal hormone relaxin and the pelvis being more moldable and malleable and able to be brought together without osteotomy. If the patient is brought to the operating room and the pelvic bones cannot be brought together easily under anesthesia, an osteotomy would be performed. The parents should be counseled that if a successful initial closure occurs and the bladder grows with time, the child has a chance of voiding and being continent from below in experienced hands, but this varies from 20% to 70%. You would tell the family that the sexual function of males with bladder exstrophy is normal and that fertility through normal procreation is very low. However, sperm can be harvested easily from the testis, and many normal babies have been delivered from males born with bladder exstrophy through in vitro fertilization. Sexual function and fertility in females with exstrophy is normal. They should know that the vagina is shorter and wider than normal and that the cervix enters the vagina in the anterior wall and not in the dome of the vagina, and thus they are more prone to uterine prolapse.

Suggested reading

Gearhart JP. The bladder exstrophy-epispadias-cloacal exstrophy complex. In: *Pediatric Urology*. 1st ed. Philadelphia: Saunders;2001:511–46.

Sponseller PD, Bisson LJ, Gearhart JP, et al. The anatomy of the pelvis in the exstrophy complex. *J Bone Joint Surg Am*. 1995;77(2):177–89.

Stec A, Pannu H, Tadros Y, et al. Evaluation of the bony pelvis in classic exstrophy by using 3D CT: further insights. *J Urol*. 2001;58:1030–35.

Stec A, Pannu H, Tadros Y, et al. Pelvic floor anatomy in classic bladder exstrophy using 3-dimensional computerized tomography: initial insights. *J Urol*. 2001;166:1444–9.

CASE 2

An obstetrician and gynecologist calls with the findings of a huge abdominal mass and a large spinal abnormality found on a late-term ultrasound done for pregnancy dates. Another ultrasound and amniocentesis show a 46,XY karyotype. Before the ultrasound arrives for your review, the baby is delivered with the findings seen in Fig. 6.2 (where the narrow arrow shows the hemiphallus and the wide arrow shows the hemibladder).

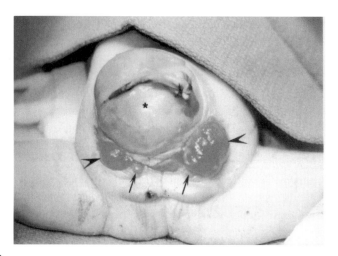

Fig. 6.2

1 How would you describe this birth defect to the family?
2 What is the incidence and sex ratio in this defect?
3 Are there bony and renal defects associated with this anomaly?
4 What would you tell the family about the need for surgery?
5 What would you tell the family about the sex of rearing and fertility?

Discussion

1 This birth defect should be described to the family as a major lower abdominal, gastrointestinal, and genitourinary defect. An omphalocele that contains varying amounts of bowel content is present, and the bladder presents on the abdominal wall in two halves with a midgut plate (ileocecal plate) between the bladder halves. There is a bifid phallus and an imperforate anus. Fifty to seventy percent of these patients also present with a spina bifida.
2 The incidence of this birth defect is 1 in 400,000 live births, and the sex ratio is 2:1 male to female.
3 Bony and neural defects in this anomaly include greater than 38% shortage of bone in the pubis and marked internal rotation of the anterior

and posterior pelvis, and 50% to 70% of the patients have neural tube defects associated with this anomaly. In addition, many have a single kidney.

4 If a major neurological defect is present, it takes precedence in the repair process. The family should be counseled that surgery should begin within the first few hours after birth. This would include a colostomy or ileostomy and joining of the bladder halves in the midline. In carefully selected patients without a major neurological defect, the bladder halves can be joined and the bladder placed in the abdomen. If possible, surgery should be done in the first few hours of life if the child is in a reasonable physiological condition. Historically, some patients with cloacal exstrophy with 46,XY karyotype have been gender-converted to females. However, recent literature shows that this may indeed not be the correct approach. However, the information is scant and no large studies exist supporting either side of this question. The histological microstructure of the testes in males with cloacal exstrophy is normal, but fertility has not been reported.

Suggested reading

Gearhart JP. The bladder exstrophy-epispadias-cloacal exstrophy complex. In: *Pediatric Urology*. 1st ed.Philadelphia: Saunders;2001:511–46.

Gearhart JP, Jeffs RD. Techniques to create urinary continence in cloacal exstrophy patients. *J Urol*. 1991;146:616–19.

Mathews R, Jeffs RD, Reiner WG, et al. Cloacal exstrophy—improving the quality of life: the Johns Hopkins experience. *J Urol*. 1998;160:2552–6.

Mathews R, Perlman E, Gearhart JP. Gonadal morphology in cloacal exstrophy: implications in gender assignment. *Br J Urol Int*. 1999;83:484–8.

Schober J, Carmichael P, Hines M, et al. The ultimate challenge of cloacal exstrophy. *J Urol*. 2002;167:300–304.

CASE 3

An infant shows up in your consulting room who is now four weeks old and came from another country with the defect seen in Fig. 6.3.

1 How would you describe this to the family?
2 What is the incidence of this defect?
3 What would you tell the infant's family about the timing of surgery?
4 What will you tell the family about eventual continence and other urinary defects?

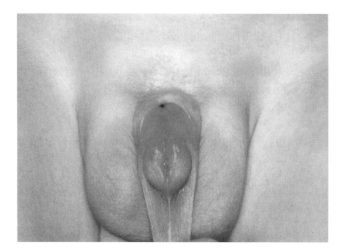

Fig. 6.3

Discussion

1 This is a complete male epispadias. The penis is short and wide with a nice urethral groove and without sphincters that keep urine inside the bladder. The penis is 50% shorter than normal and 30% wider than normal.

2 The incidence of this birth defect is 1 in 117,000 live male births.

3 The urethra should be closed and the penis reconstructed anytime between 6 and 12 months of age.

4 An eventual outlet procedure to render the child continent of urine should be performed around the age of 4–5 years, when the bladder has grown to sufficient size and the child is ready to undergo a continence procedure. Also, 50% to 60% of these children have vesicoureteral reflux, and this would be corrected at the time of an outlet procedure. Eventual continence in this group of patients is better than in the exstrophy group. If the bladder grows appropriately and these children have an appropriate outlet procedure, fully 75% to 80% of them can be rendered continent of urine when they grow older.

Suggested reading

Gearhart JP. The bladder exstrophy-epispadias-cloacal exstrophy complex. In: *Pediatric Urology*. 1st ed.Philadelphia: Saunders;2001:511–46.

Kajbafzadeh A, Duffy PG, Ransley PG. The evolution of penile reconstruction and epispadias repair: a report of 180 cases. *J Urol*. 1995;154:858–61.

Surer I, Baker L, Jeffs RD, Gearhart JP. The modified Cantwell-Ransley repair in exstrophy and epispadias: 10 year experience. *J Urol*. 2000;164:1040–4.

CASE 4

This child, referred from the general practitioner (GP)/pediatrician, shows up in your consulting room with a complaint of "never a dry nappie." On examination the findings are seen (Fig. 6.4).

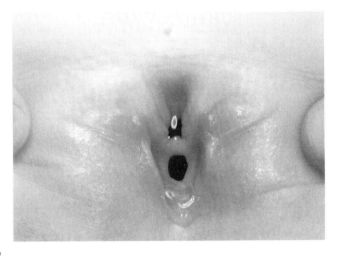

Fig. 6.4

1 In your consultant's letter, what do you tell the GP about this birth defect?
2 What do you tell the family about the timing of surgery and eventual continence?
3 What do you tell the family about sexual function and fertility?

Discussion

1 This is a female epispadias. In your consultant's letter you should inform the GP/pediatrician that this is a very rare birth defect occurring in 1 of 400,000 live births. There is a bifid clitoris, and there is no urethra and only a large cleft in the midline where the urethra should be. Furthermore, if the child pushes and coughs and there is a pink structure coming from between the legs, this is the anterior surface of the bladder.
2 The child will need the external genitalia and the urethra reconstructed in order to increase bladder outlet resistance and to make the bladder grow. The timing of surgery should be around 6 months to 1 year of age, when the urethra can be closed and the genitalia repaired. Continence can occur if the bladder grows to a sufficient size, and the child can have an appropriate outlet procedure at 4–5 years of age when she is ready to be continent. Continence rates are 70% to 80%.

3 You can reassure the family that the child's sexual function and fertility will be normal. The vagina is shorter and wider than normal, but this does not hinder sexual function, orgasm, or fertility.

Suggested reading

Gearhart JP. The bladder exstrophy-epispadias-cloacal exstrophy complex. In: *Pediatric Urology*. 1st ed. Philadelphia: Saunders;2001:511–46.

Gearhart JP, Peppas DS, Jeffs RD. Complete genitourinary reconstruction in female epispadias. *J Urol*. 1993;149(5):1110–13.

Hendren WW. Congenital female epispadias with incontinence. *J Urol*. 1981;125:558–62.

7 | Vesicoureteric Reflux

Pierre Mouriquand

CASE 1

Tracy is a 7-year-old girl who is referred by her general practitioner (GP) for recurrent episodes of febrile urinary tract infections (UTIs) and occasional diurnal urinary incontinence.

1 Why is taking the medical history of this child so important?
2 Is there a need to organize investigations, and which ones?
3 What advice would you give to the parents?
4 Is there a place for radical treatments of reflux in this situation?

Discussion

1 Taking the medical history tells you in most cases why this little girl meets with this problem.

Tracy does not like to go to the toilets at school because they are dirty and hates sitting on them. Hence she waits until the last minute when her bladder is screaming to be emptied. When she goes to the toilet, she does not sit on the seat and she empties her bladder by pushing to shorten her stay in that unpleasant place. She also pulls her trousers down at the level of her knees, and so she empties her bladder with her two thighs together. This unsatisfactory position facilitates intravaginal reflux of urine. All the ingredients are there to explain her symptoms: (i) She does not go regularly to the toilets and tends to wait until she is at home to void in better conditions. Hence urine stays a very long time in the bladder. (ii) She pushes to pass water because she wants to shorten her stay in these dirty toilets and has a position over the toilet bowl that does not allow to relax her muscles to achieve a complete bladder emptying. She therefore keeps a urine residue after each micturition, which facilitates infections. (iii) She has intravaginal reflux of urine, which may facilitate infections as well. (iv) Moreover, she avoids drinking to avoid going to the toilets. Her urine is concentrated and the restricting fluid also aggravates her chronic constipation, which is an important additional factor inducing recurrent UTIs. Once you have detected the underlying problem, you also need to make sure that this girl does not have serious family or school disorders such as violence or sexual abuse that could be expressed by urological symptoms (Hinman syndrome). Clinical examination should include palpation of the abdomen (constipation), examination of her genitalia (abnormal meatus, signs of violence), and examination of her spine and feet to detect a possible underlying neurological disorder (sacral pit).

2 Although the situation seems to be straightforward, several complementary investigations are needed to rule out underlying urological anomalies.

A plain abdominal X-ray gives you three main pieces of information. It shows (i) the overloaded bowels, (ii) possible urinary stones (unlikely in Western children), and (iii) an abnormal spine, which can be associated with neurological disorders.

A pre- and postmicturition ultrasound scan of the urinary tract may show you (i) a dilated urinary tract reflecting a urine flow impairment (UFI) or less likely a dilated upper urinary tract caused by reflux, (ii) a postmicturition residue, and (iii) a thick-walled bladder.

A micturating cystogram using contrast is also recommended and may show you a vesicoureteric reflux, irregular bladder walls, and a classical spinningtop appearance of the urethra during micturition, which reflects vesicosphincteric dyssynergia (Tracy pushes to pass water and therefore contracts her perineal muscles, which creates an outlet obstruction and causes postmicturition urine residue).

Three to 6 months after the last episode of febrile UTI, a DMSA scan can be organized to exclude any renal damage caused by infection. In Tracy's case, the DMSA scan is normal.

3 Very clearly, Tracy does not use her bladder and bowels properly. The reflux (uni- or bilateral) is most likely secondary to the abnormal urodynamic bladder profile. It is a so-called low-grade reflux, i.e. it is unlikely to cause an ultrasound distension of the upper urinary tract. The reflux in Tracy's case is a "symptom" and not a "disease" in itself. It is therefore essential to correct the bladder and bowel dysfunctions by giving the right advice. Tracy should regularly go to the toilet every 2–3 hours during the day. She should sit on the toilet, pull her trousers down to the ankles so she can open her legs, and relax her abdominal and perineal muscles. She should also spend enough time on the toilet to empty her bladder completely without pushing. She should understand that passing water and passing a stool are two different actions. The first implies relaxing her muscles, whereas the second implies contracting her abdominal muscles.

Constipation should be actively treated by giving dietary advice and a 3-month course of lactulose.

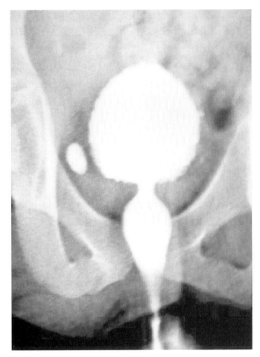

Fig. 7.1 Cystography showing vesicosphincteric dyssynergia (spinningtop urethra), irregular bladder walls, and a small bladder diverticulum.

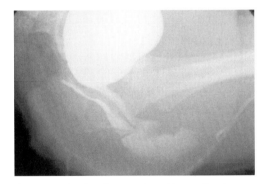

Fig. 7.2 Cystography: vaginal reflux during micturition and vesicoureteric reflux.

Because of the vesicoureteric reflux, a 3-month course of antibioprophylaxis can be given until Tracy changes her habits. There is however low evidence that antibioprophylaxis is useful to prevent UTIs. Because the DMSA scan is normal and because the bladder behavior is going to improve, it is most likely that the reflux will disappear with time.

4 There are however cases like Tracy's where a radical correction of the vesicoureteric reflux might be considered. If Tracy continues to get febrile UTIs despite all your very good advice and treatment, or if repeated DMSA scans demonstrate a deterioration of the renal parenchyma, it is accepted that a correction of reflux might be advisable. This can either be done by open surgery or by injecting a biocompatible substance under the refluxing ureteric orifice. However, correcting the underlying functional disorder remains the first priority, and good result of surgery cannot be expected if the bladder and bowels habits remain inadequate. The choice between open surgery and endoscopic treatment varies from one center to another. It is acknowledged that open surgery provides better long-term results in terms of curing the reflux than endoscopic treatments.

CASE 2

Five years later, you see Tracy again; she has just started her periods. Although she is well and free of UTIs, she comes back to your outpatient department with a new micturating cystography showing that the reflux is unchanged.
1 What would you do?

Discussion

The most accepted current attitude is to ignore this reflux and simply ask Tracy to check her urine bacteriology each time she is febrile. Others are anxious that in a few years' time Tracy will start her sexual life, will get pregnant, and might be more exposed to UTIs. They would therefore advocate stopping the reflux in order to put her kidneys in a safer situation. The validity of this attitude has not been shown to date.

CASE 3

John is 5 months old and was born with an antenatal history of dilated upper urinary tracts detected at the end of gestation. He is otherwise fit and healthy. A postnatal ultrasound scan and a cystography were performed at 2 days of life to exclude posterior urethral valves. This confirmed a marked dilatation of both ureters and pelves and slightly echogenic parenchymas on both sides. The cystography showed a massive vesicoureteric reflux on both sides, no

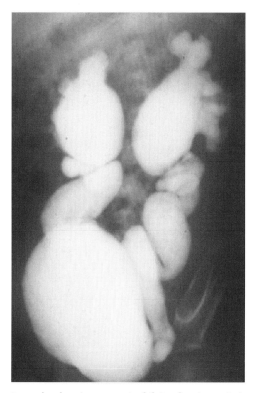

Fig. 7.3 John's cystography showing a massive bilateral vesicoureteric reflux.

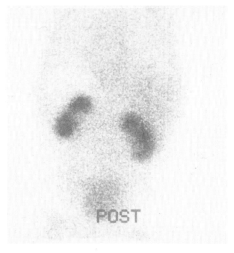

Fig. 7.4 John's DMSA scan showing bilateral heterogeneous renal parenchymas.

urethral valves, and a normal-looking bladder (Fig. 7.3). A DMSA scan performed 6 weeks after birth showed bilaterally damaged kidneys with a 38% relative function to the left and 62% to the right kidney (Fig. 7.4).

John was put on prophylactic antibiotics, and he made very good progress until 3 days ago when he developed a febrile UTI.

1 What should you do?

2 Would you screen his two brothers and his sister for reflux?

Discussion

1 John was born with a bilateral severe vesicoureteric reflux suspected antenatally after the dilatation of both ureters and pelves. Fifteen percent of antenatal dilatations of the urinary tract are related to reflux (vs. 50% related to an abnormal urine flow at the level of the pyelouretic junction). From birth onward, he was put on chemoprophylaxis to prevent the risk of UTI, which is knowingly increased in patients with reflux. The DMSA scan performed at 6 weeks of age confirmed that the renal substance is abnormal in both kidneys. Around 50% of children with an early diagnosis of reflux have an abnormal DMSA. This is not an acquired damage of the parenchyma caused by a UTI (i.e. "reflux nephropathy"), but it is a congenital structural anomaly of the renal substance due to its abnormal development (i.e. dysplasia). You first need to check the bacteriology report with the antibiogram, which shows that the trimethoprim you initially prescribed does not work on this *Escherichia coli* infection. (i) You put him on amoxicillin for 10 days. (ii) You therefore adjust the antibiotherapy. In many European centers, John is admitted to a children's ward to receive intravenous antibiotherapy, which usually combines a third-generation cephalosporin and an aminoglycoside. (iii) After curing his febrile infection, you discharge John from hospital and let him go home with an antibioprophylaxis adjusted to the antibiogram.

2 Around 30% of siblings of children with reflux present with vesicoureteric reflux, most of them being completely asymptomatic. Considering that contrast cystography is a rather invasive procedure (urethral catheter, irradiations, morbidity) and that ultrasonography is of little help for the positive diagnosis of vesicoureteric reflux, most centers would not screen asymptomatic siblings. It may be that the most sensible investigation to prescribe in the siblings would be a DMSA scan, which, if it is normal, would be completely reassuring because even if there is reflux, the chances to see it going with growth are very high. On the other hand, if it is abnormal a specific follow-up would be organized.

CASE 4

Three months later, John presented with another febrile UTI despite his new antibioprophylaxis.

1 What should you do?

Discussion

1 Obviously, conservative management is not successful in John's case and alternative treatments need to be considered: (i) A radical correction of reflux in an 8-month-old baby presenting with a bilateral massive reflux is a difficult procedure because the bladder is small and the ureters are very big. If this option was chosen, it is most likely that a ureteric modeling would be performed; this procedure has a significant morbidity. Moreover, the neurologic behavior of the bladder changes a lot during the first year of life, and it may be damaging for these neurologic events to perform an operation that implies a rather extensive dissection of the trigonal region. For these various reasons, ureteric reimplantation is not considered a first option in this situation. (ii) A second option would be to stop reflux by injecting a biocompatible substance (Macroplastique/Deflux) behind the intramural ureter in order to increase its backing and restore the antireflux mechanisms. Although less invasive in terms of neurologic threat, this option remains quite aggressive in an 8-month toddler with a small urethra. Considering the severity of John's reflux, it is also likely that this injection would have a poor chance of success. (iii) Therefore the idea of stopping the reflux to protect the upper tracts at this age does not seem to be the most appropriate approach, and it might be more sensible to reduce the risk of UTIs by removing the prepuce, which is a well-known reservoir of bacteria in boys. Although there are no published controlled studies demonstrating that circumcision is an efficient way to reduce UTIs, much data seems to reinforce this approach. This is the option chosen in John's case.

CASE 5

John is now 24 months and almost potty trained and has done quite well since his last consultation. However, he presented last week with another febrile UTI, which was adequately treated by the GP.

1 Are there any investigations you wish to organize at this point, and why?

2 Considering that reflux persists, would you plan a radical correction of the reflux?

3 What surgical options do you have?

4 How would you follow up this child?

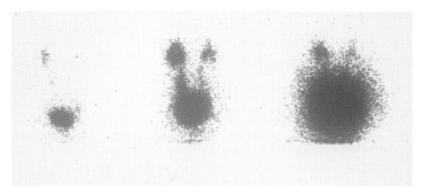

Fig. 7.5 Direct isotope cystography. *Source:* Godley, 2001.

Discussion

1 John's situation has changed. His bladder has matured and he has reasonable control of his micturition. It would be helpful to know if the reflux
is still there and if the recent febrile UTI has caused any parenchymal
damage.

   Standard contrast cystography, indirect isotope cystography, and direct
isotope cystography are the three options available to check if the reflux
is still present. The contrast study remains the standard in most places
although it implies a bladder catheterization and a significant exposure
to radiation. Indirect isotope cystography focuses on an increase of ra-
dioactivity in the renal regions during micturition. It avoids a bladder
catheterization and provides much less radiation than contrast cystography. However, it is much less sensitive than the other two techniques and
can miss a significant reflux. Direct isotope cystography does not avoid urethral catheterization but has also a low radiation rate. It is a very sensitive,
probably the best, test to detect reflux although it does not give you clear
data on the anatomy of the lower urinary tract. This is the investigation
you choose in John's case, and it shows a persistent massive vesicoureteric
reflux (Fig. 7.5).

   The second investigation that will be useful in your decision is a new
DMSA scan, which should tell you if the situation has changed since
the initial scan. This test should not be organized too soon after the last
febrile UTI as there are intraparenchymal inflammatory reactions that
accompany UTIs and disappear within 3 months. Hence John needs a new
DMSA scan 3–6 months after the last UTI. This scan still shows bilateral
parenchymal heterogeneity with a possible aggravation of a defect in the
upper pole of the left kidney. The relative function of the left kidney has
gone down to 31%. The interpretation of this change of function is difficult,

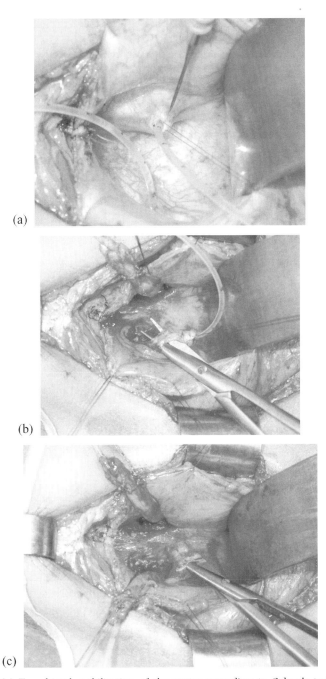

Fig. 7.6 (a) Transhiatal mobilization of the ureter according to Cohen's technique. (b) Freeing of both ureters in John's case. (c) Both ureters are free. The tip of the Reynolds scissors is lifting the bladder mucosa to create the submucosal tunnel. (*Continued p. 84.*)

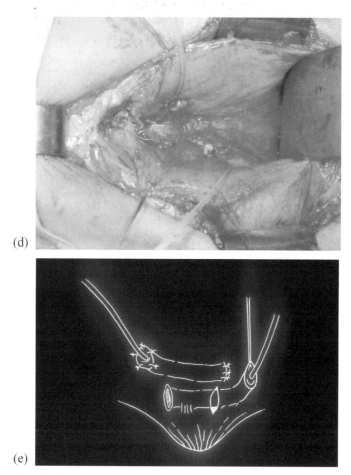

(d)

(e)

Fig. 7.6 (Contd.) (d) Both ureters are sitting under a submucosa tunnel, the left ureter below the right in this particular case. (e) Transtrigonal ureteric reimplantation according to Cohen's technique.

as it may correspond either to a real decrease of the relative function of the left kidney or to a more marked development of the right kidney.

2 Persistent symptomatic UTIs despite well-conducted antibioprophylaxis and decrease of relative renal function are the two main indications of radical correction of vesicoureteric reflux. Hence, in John's case, you feel it is appropriate to correct the reflux. The parents should know that the aim of this treatment is only to stop reflux and that it will not have any effect on the number of UTIs and on the present renal damage. However, it is established that correcting reflux reduces the risk of upper tract UTIs and pyelonephritis. This is the reason that you feel appropriate to correct this reflux.

3 To stop reflux you can either propose an open procedure or an endoscopic procedure. Endoscopic treatments have the best results in low-grade refluxes, which, in most cases, do not require any radical treatment as they usually reflect an underlying functional disorder (see table). The percentage of success of biocompatible substances in severe reflux is disappointing compared with that of open surgery. In John's case, there is little doubt that an open ureteric reimplantation is the best option. There are several techniques to reimplant the ureters. (i) The transhiatal procedures (mainly the

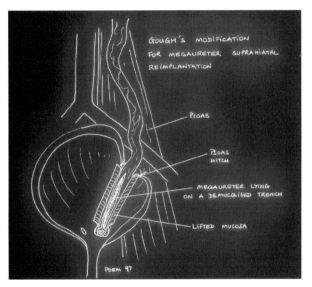

Fig. 7.7 Gough's modification of the suprahiatal reimplantation of the ureter in case of megaureter.

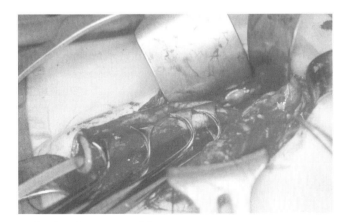

Fig. 7.8 Hendren's technique to model the ureter.

Cohen's procedure) consist in dissecting the transmural ureter from inside the bladder, freeing it, and repositioning it under a tunnel of mucosa across the trigone (Fig. 7.6 a–e). (ii) The suprahiatal reimplantation consists in freeing the ureter outside the bladder and reinsert it in the bladder under a tunnel of mucosa using a different point of entry. This allows to get a longer tunnel, which extends from the upper posterior part of the bladder down to the trigone. This is the technique of choice with large ureters where a transtrigonal reimplantation would not allow an antireflux system to be achieved (Fig. 7.7). It is necessary to create a length of submucosal tunnel at least 4 times the diameter of the reimplanted ureter to obtain an antireflux system (Paquin). In some cases, the ureter is too big to be reimplanted and needs to be modeled to get a satisfactory caliber (Hendren's technique or folding techniques) (Fig. 7.8). (iii) The Gregoir Lich technique consists of lengthening the submucosal segment of ureter via an extravesical dissection. It may jeopardize the nerves going to the bladder, and bilateral reimplantation is not recommended in one procedure. (iv) The Jill Vernet technique is more applicable for low-grade refluxes. It consists of bringing together the two ureteric orifices by attracting them toward the midline. In John's case the two ureters are big; this necessitates a suprahiatal reimplantation.

4 Although the operation you performed was very successful in terms of stopping the bilateral vesicoureteric reflux, John needs a close follow-up of his severe uronephrologic malformation. From the nephrologic point of view, both parenchymas are damaged and some scars may continue to progress although the reflux is cured and John no longer has febrile UTIs. Regular checks of his blood pressure and microalbuminuria are advisable. When he reaches puberty, the nephrologists may discuss a more detailed assessment of his renal functions. From the urologic point of view, an assessment of the dilatation of the ureters by an ultrasound scan is advisable 3 months after the ureteric reimplantation. A persistent dilatation is often found, but it should slowly decrease with time. Some surgeons like to check that the reflux has gone and that the renal function remains stable or slightly improves by performing a Mag 3 scan with an indirect cystography 6 months after surgery. There is no consensus on the need of keeping the child on prophylactic antibiotics for a few months after surgery.

Conclusions

Tracy and John's cases are very different and the table below attempts to give the main features of the "reflux-symptoms" and the "reflux-disease".

	VUR symptom	VUR disease
Sex	Essentially girls	Essentially boys
Antenatal diagnosis	No	Yes
Ultrasonography	No dilatation	Dilatation
Grade	≤ 3	≥ 3
DMSA	Normal	Abnormal $> 50\%$
Cessation rate	High	$< 50\%$
Cause	Lower tract dysfunction	Malformation
Treatment	Reeducation	Surgery
Incidence	$++++++$	$++$

There is a grey zone between these two categories of reflux where difficulties occur to define the best management. The main current controversies about reflux concern the need of chemoprophylaxis and its duration, the time and place of radical treatments, the indications for endoscopic treatments, and the relation between reflux and UTIs.

Suggested reading

Godley ML. Vesicoureteral reflux: pathophysiology and experimental studies. In: Gearhart JP, Rink RC, Mouriquand P, eds. *Pediatric Urology*. Philadelphia: Saunders; 2001:359–81.

Greenfield SP, Wan J. The diagnosis and medical management of primary vesicoureteral reflux. In: Gearhart JP, Rink RC, Mouriquand P, eds. *Pediatric Urology*. Philadelphia: Saunders; 2001:382–410.

Park JM, Retik AB. Surgery for vesicoureteral reflux. In: Gearhart JP, Rink RC, Mouriquand P, eds. *Pediatric Urology*. Philadelphia: Saunders; 2001:421–9.

Puri P. Endoscopic treatment of vesicoureteral reflux. In: Gearhart JP, Rink RC, Mouriquand P, eds. *Pediatric Urology*. Philadelphia: Saunders; 2001:411–20.

Yeung CK. Pathophysiology of bladder dysfunction. In: Gearhart JP, Rink RC, Mouriquand P, eds. *Pediatric Urology*. Philadelphia: Saunders; 2001:453–69.

8 | Congenital Anomalies of the Kidney and Ureter

Stuart O'Toole

Introduction

The complex embryologic origins of the renal tract ensure that there are a large number of congenital abnormalities of the kidney and ureter. The advent of antenatal ultrasound has resulted in the majority of these abnormalities presenting at a stage when they are asymptomatic. The evidence for the postnatal management of these problems is at best patchy. This means that the management of these infants and children vary widely between clinicians. The following four cases have been picked to illustrate some common clinical scenarios that present to the pediatric urologist.

CASE 1

A normal, full-term infant presents with an antenatal diagnosis of a right-sided cystic kidney. The contralateral kidney looked normal on the antenatal ultrasound, and the pregnancy was otherwise uncomplicated. The postnatal ultrasound suggested a multicystic dysplastic kidney (MCDK) (Fig. 8.1) with an entirely normal-looking contralateral kidney.

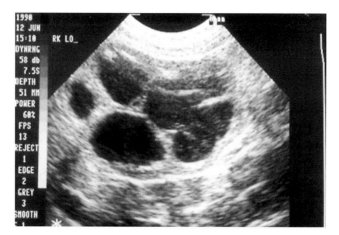

Fig. 8.1 Postnatal ultrasound showing a multicystic dysplastic kidney.

1 What further investigations are required?

2 The parents have seen a television program that suggested that these kidneys can cause problems and should be removed with keyhole surgery. What do you advise them?

Discussion

1 An MCDK should have no function; therefore to confirm this diagnosis a technetium-labeled dimercaptosuccinic acid (DMSA) or dimercaptoacetyltriglycine (MAG3) scan should be performed. It is not uncommon for a grossly hydronephrotic kidney secondary to a pelviureteric junction (PUJ) obstruction to be diagnosed antenatally as MCDK, and so a functional study is mandatory.

Vesicoureteric reflux has been reported in 20–40% of the infants with MCDK. Many clinicians therefore feel that a micturating cystourethrogam (MCUG) is also necessary. Other clinicians counter with a more conservative approach. They argue that in the presence of a normal ultrasound, the incidence of reflux is reduced and the reflux itself is of a low grade and should resolve with time. MCUG itself is an invasive test with its own incidence of complications. If this less invasive approach is taken, then the decision not to do an MCUG should be taken in conjunction with the parents. The primary care physician should also be made aware of the possibility of reflux, and any unexplained febrile illness should be taken seriously.

2 With the advent of new technology and less invasive surgical techniques, it is sometimes tempting to change the indications for a procedure. An MCDK can be removed easily via a laparoscopic approach, and the surgical insult to the child is minimal. However, all procedures carry risk and we should evaluate the current evidence for the removal of an asymptomatic MCDK.

Prior to the advent of antenatal ultrasound, MCDK was thought to be exceptionally rare and tended to present as an abdominal mass. The current incidence is now much higher than previously thought and ranges between 1 in 3000 and 1 in 4000. If these kidneys are simply observed from birth, then a number of them will decrease in size or involute spontaneously. A recent series reported a rate of involution of 52% at a median age of 6.5 years.

Nephrectomy has been advocated by some in children with MCDK, because of the risk of developing malignancy or hypertension. Manzone and Caldamone reviewed the literature over a 30-year period and found just 12 cases of malignancy associated with MCDK, 6 of which were Wilms tumours. In the same review they uncovered 13 cases of hypertension, 11 of which responded to removing the MCDK.

It would therefore seem that the risk of developing complications from MCDK is relatively small, probably much less than 1 in 1000 cases. Even though a nephrectomy is safe and well tolerated by a child, most clinicians believe that there is not sufficient evidence to advocate it routinely. It would therefore seem reasonable that in an infant with a definitive diagnosis of MCDK a conservative policy of observation should be adopted. This can be achieved with ultrasound and yearly measurement of blood pressure.

In my own practice, nephrectomy is reserved for children with diagnostic difficulties or those who have an enlarging MCDK on follow-up. This is achieved laparoscopically using a retroperitoneal approach with a minimal hospital stay.

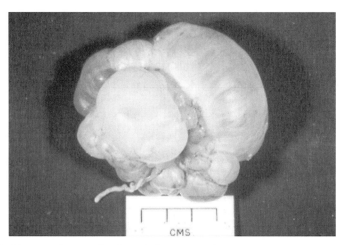

Fig. 8.2 A large multicystic dysplastic kidney removed at open operation.

Suggested reading

Belk RA, Thomas DF, Mueller RF, et al. A family study and the natural history of prenatally detected unilateral multicystic dysplastic kidney. *J Urol.* Feb. 2002;167(2 pt 1): 666–9.

Manzoni GM, Caldamone AA. Multicystic kidney. In: Stringer MD, Oldham KT, Mouriquand PDE, Howard ER, eds. *Paediatric Surgery and Urology: Long Term Outcome.* London: Saunders;1998:632–41.

CASE 2

A 6-week-old boy presents with an antenatal diagnosis of left-sided hy-dronephrosis. The presence of hydronephrosis with hydroureter has been confirmed by postnatal ultrasound examination (Fig. 8.3), and the child has been started on antibiotic prophylaxis.

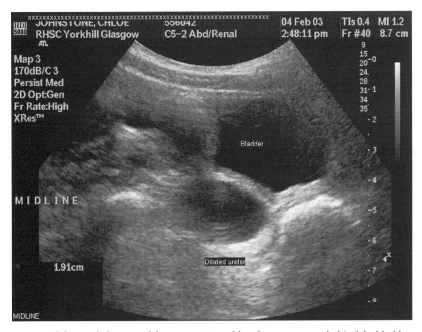

Fig. 8.3 Abdominal ultrasound demonstrating a dilated ureter present behind the bladder.

1 What are the possible diagnoses, and what further investigations are re-quired? What is the natural history of this condition?

2 What are the indications for surgery?

3 Which surgery should be performed?

4 When should the surgery be performed?

Discussion

1 This young boy has presented with a megaureter. This is a descriptive term for a dilated ureter with or without pelvicalyceal dilation. This label does not indicate the cause of the dilation.

The ureter can be:

- refluxing;
- obstructed;

- refluxing and obstructed;
- nonobstructed and nonrefluxing.

The megaureter can be secondary to bladder outflow obstruction, infection, external compression, or a neuropathic bladder. Commonly, no causative problem can be identified; in this case it is referred to as a primary megaureter.

The megaureter can be quite easily diagnosed on ultrasound. A physical examination should be performed to look for any congenital anomalies that may predispose to the presence of a neuropathic bladder (e.g. spina bifida, sacral agenesis). An MCUG should also be performed; it will be able to exclude the presence of bladder outflow obstruction and demonstrate if the megaureter is due to reflux or not. The diagnosis of obstruction is much more problematic, especially in the small child with a large megaureter. Diuretic renography is normally used, but care should be taken in the interpretation of the results, because it is difficult to distinguish between a truly obstructed system and a dilated system. Occasionally, a retrograde or antegrade study may be required (Fig. 8.4). In the case illustrated no vesicoureteric reflux was demonstrated during the MCUG, which raised the possibility of a primary obstructed megaureter. The diuretic renogram illustrated some holdup at the vesicoureteric junction (VUJ); the report raised the possibility of obstruction, but could not confirm it.

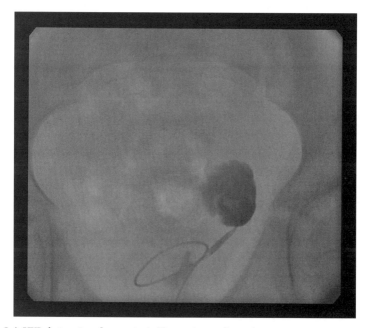

Fig. 8.4 VUJ obstruction demonstrated by a retrograde study.

2 A child with an unobstructed primary megaureter would be expected to have normal kidneys and is unlikely to require any active management. Historically, a child with an obstructed megaureter would have presented with symptoms and would have been managed by surgery. However, infants now present antenatally, with obstructed primary megaureters. These infants are often entirely asymptomatic with kidneys that are functioning well. In the literature, there are a number of examples of these infants being treated conservatively. The majority of these hydroureters appear to resolve with conservative management, and only a small number (approximately a fifth) requiring surgery. There is some suggestion from literature that a ureter measuring greater than 10 mm is less likely to resolve spontaneously.

3 There are four established indications for surgery in a primary obstructed megaureter:
- A decrease in function of the kidney during follow-up.
- An increase in the size of the hydroureter on serial ultrasound.
- Symptoms of infection or pain.
- Urolithiasis.

Other authors advocate surgery if the ureter is particularly large or there is decreased function in the kidney at presentation.

4 The definitive surgical treatment for a primary obstructed megaureter is excision of the narrow segment and reimplantation of the ureter using an antireflux procedure. The Leadbetter-Politano or Cohen techniques are most commonly used for reimplantation. It is generally accepted that the length of the tunnel should be 5 times the width of the ureter. Most authors recommend tapering ureters that are wider than 10 mm when decompressed.

5 Tapering and reimplantation of a ureter is a major undertaking in a small bladder. It is therefore advisable to delay this type of surgery until the child is at least 6 months of age. Most authors would recommend delaying surgery until 1 year of age. If more urgent surgery is required, then a cutaneous ureterostomy is the standard technique although this makes subsequent reconstruction more troublesome. As an alternative, it is possible to place a JJ stent across the VUJ via open cystostomy. This technique has been advocated by Ransley as a temporizing measure, but it can lead to permanent resolution of the obstruction (personal communication).

A child with a diagnosis of primary megaureter can provide a diagnostic and management challenge. A stepwise and logical approach will be required for diagnosis. In most cases a conservative strategy of careful observation, coupled with timely surgery if required, is the management of choice.

Suggested reading

Liu HY, Dhillon HK, Yeung CK, Diamond DA, Duffy PG, Ransley PG. Clinical outcome and management of prenatally diagnosed primary megaureters. *J Urol.* Aug. 1994;152 614.

CASE 3

A 10-week-old baby presented with pyrexia and was systemically unwell. She was being treated for a urinary tract infection after a coliform organism had been cultured from a suprapubic aspirate. General examination revealed a toxic child with a bulging mass visible at the introitus (Fig. 8.5).

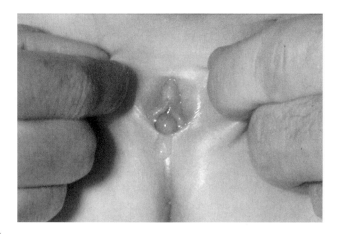

Fig. 8.5

1 What is the differential diagnosis?
2 What is the immediate management?
3 What other investigations are required?
4 If this infant had presented antenatally, how should she have been managed?

Discussion

1 Although this particular child presented with an ectopic ureterocele, the diagnosis could have been one of an imperforate hymen or a paraurethral cyst. In this case a diagnosis could be made on the basis of an ultrasound examination although in both an imperforate hymen and a prolapsing ureterocele one could expect bladder outlet obstruction and bilateral

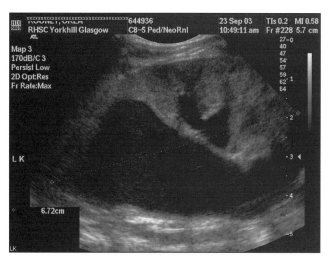

Fig. 8.6 Ultrasound of left kidney showing a dilated upper moiety in a duplex kidney.

hydronephrosis. The ultrasound in this case demonstrated a degree of bilateral hydronephrosis with a left-sided duplex system (Fig. 8.6). The ultrasound of the pelvis did not show a hydrometrocolpos.

2 A child with an infected ureterocele that is both prolapsing and causing obstruction can be extremely unwell. If the child can be stabilized and resuscitated, then it may be possible to take the child to theater and incise the ureterocele cystoscopically. At cystosopy, the incision of the ureterocele should be made close to the bladder wall to minimize the risk of upper pole reflux subsequently. However, if the child is too unwell for surgery, then the prolapsed portion of the ureterocele can be punctured at the bedside and a urethral catheter inserted. This maneuver permits drainage of the infected upper tract and also allows bladder drainage.

3 A prolapsing ureterocele is almost always associated with a duplex kidney ipsilaterally. The ureter from the upper moiety of a duplex kidney is inserted more caudally than normal and is prone to obstruction at the level of the VUJ. The lower moiety ureter is often inserted more laterally and is prone to vesicoureteric reflux. As either of the moieties can be functioning poorly in a duplex system, it is advisable to perform both an MCUG and a DMSA scan (Fig. 8.7). If diagnostic difficulty remains, then intravenous urography or magnetic resonance imaging (MRI) urography may beneficial.

The majority of babies with a ureterocele and duplex kidneys present antenatally. When seen by the pediatric urologist, they are usually asymptomatic. The management of a child who is acutely unwell is relatively standardized. Most pediatric urologists would puncture the

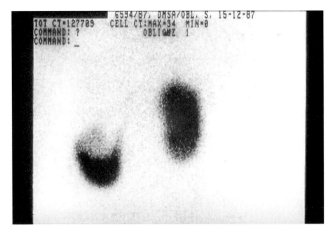

Fig. 8.7 DMSA scan demonstrating a nonfunctioning upper moiety in a duplex kidney.

ureterocele as described above. However, there is considerable debate over what is the optimum management for the asymptomatic infant. The management options are influenced by the function of both the upper and the lower poles, the size of the ureterocele, the degree of hydronephrosis, and the presence of reflux to the lower moiety. Some of the more common presentations and surgical options are illustrated below.

Management options for a ureterocele complicating a duplex kidney

1 Conservative treatment.
2 Endoscopic incision of the ureterocele.
3 Upper pole heminephrectomy.
4 Upper pole heminephrectomy with excision of ureter and ureterocele.
5 Reimplantation of both ureters, with repair of the ureterocele.
6 Pyelopyelostomy.

Good upper pole function

There is a good case for managing these infants with just observation. If the ureterocele is large or there is significant hydronephrosis associated, then it may be punctured endoscopically. If there is a good lower pole with no vesicoureteric reflux, then a pyelopyelostomy could be appropriate. If there is symptomatic reflux into the lower moiety, then excision of the ureterocele and implantation of both ureters may be required. This, however, is not an easy operation and should be reserved for the experienced pediatric urologist.

Poor upper pole function

It is reasonable to manage some of these children by observation if there is not a significant hydronephrosis. Some pediatric urologists advocate endoscopic puncture; however, others are concerned that you run the risk of introducing reflux, which may complicate further management. If surgery is warranted due to the degree of hydronephrosis, then many pediatric urologists would recommend an upper pole heminephrectomy. This is termed the simplified approach. Here, the ureterocele is decompressed from above, and surgery within the bladder is avoided unless absolutely necessary.

A child who presents with a ureterocele provides an interesting challenge to the pediatric urologist. The anatomy and function of the system vary considerably between children, and so no one management plan is suitable for all cases. It is important to bear in mind that in these children it is always possible to injure the bladder neck or damage a perfectly normal lower pole.

Suggested reading

Mackie GG, Stephens FD. Duplex kidneys: a correlation with renal dysplasia with position of ureteric orifice. *J Urol.* Aug. 1975;114(2):274–80.

CASE 4

A 6-month-old boy is referred with an antenatal diagnosis of hydronephrosis. The referring pediatrician is concerned that the dilation of the renal pelvis has worsened during follow-up, the AP diameter (i.e. the anterior posterior diameter of the renal pelvis in the transverse plane of the kidney) having increased from 18 mm shortly after birth to 28 mm at 4 months of age. The infant has a normal MCUG. A MAG3 diuretic renogram has demonstrated poor drainage, but with a function of 51% in the affected kidney.

1 What action is required?
2 Why did this happen?
3 How can it be managed now?
4 Can ultrasound appearances predict the future requirement for surgery?
5 What are the indications for surgery?

Discussion

1 For the past 20 years, antenatal diagnosis of renal tract dilation has been a source of controversy in pediatric urology. The problem is, when is a kidney simply dilated? And when is it obstructed? If it is only dilated, then over

a period of time its function will remain the same; if it is obstructed, then the function will eventually deteriorate. In this case a child who appeared to have a degree of PUJ obstruction has shown a marked increase in his hydronephrosis in a relatively short period of time. The diuretic renogram has also shown obstruction, but with preserved function.

The work of Ransley et al. in the late 1980s demonstrated that the majority of children with this presentation and preserved function were not obstructed and could be safely followed conservatively. In the long run, the majority of the children that he followed up did not require surgery. However, the element of this presentation, which raised concern, was the deterioration in ultrasound appearances in the kidney over a relatively short period of time.

2 The main problem with this referral was that the antenatal findings were omitted from the clinical history. In this particular infant the degree of hydronephrosis present at 30 weeks of gestation was 30 mm and at 36 weeks of gestation was 28 mm. The postnatal ultrasound was done within the first few days after delivery. As the urine output in the immediate postnatal period is often lower than normal, ultrasounds at this time can underestimate the degree of hydronephrosis. When we review all of the ultrasounds performed on this infant, we can see that this kidney has remained remarkably stable over the past 9 months.

3 As this child has preserved function, it is reasonable to follow him up conservatively with regular ultrasound coupled with functional studies.

4 Dhillon et al. have methodically followed a cohort of children with hydronephrosis and presumed PUJ obstruction presenting to Great Ormond Street Hospital. The indications for surgery were the development of symptoms or a drop in ipsilateral renal function on isotope studies. Both the degree of calyceal dilatation and the AP diameter of the renal pelvis predicted the need for surgery.

AP renal pelvic diameter (mm)	Requirement for surgery (%)
>50	100
>40	80
>30	55
>20	20
<20	3

Most pediatric urologists have a cutoff point for the degree of dilation that would indicate the need for surgical intervention in their practice. It varies slightly with the age of the patient and the ease with which it is possible to follow up the patient. A dedicated unit, which has the facilities to perform isotope renograms on a regular basis, may decide to be more conservative. A unit without these facilities, dealing with a population spread over a wide geographic area, may opt to be more surgically aggressive.

5 The indications for surgery in this child are the development of symptoms (e.g. pain, infection, or stones), a drop in function of the affected kidney, and progression of the hydronephrosis. This child was followed up regularly

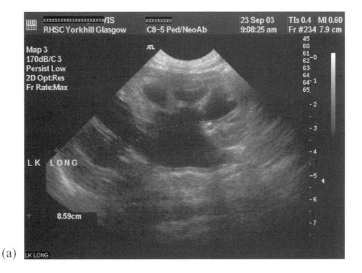

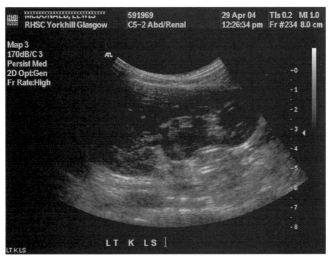

Fig. 8.8 Ultrasound of a kidney illustrating a PUJ obstruction (a) before and (b) after pyeloplasty.

for 3 years, and his imaging demonstrated a gradual improvement in both ultrasound appearance and drainage on isotope renography. However, at the age of 5 years he started to develop nonspecific symptoms of abdominal pain. His ultrasound demonstrated deterioration in hydronephrosis; and his diuretic renogram showed preserved function, but with an obstructed curve. An Anderson Hynes dismembered pyeloplasty was therefore performed, which led to resolution of his hydronephrosis and a cure for his abdominal pain (Fig. 8.8).

In managing a child with a potential PUJ obstruction, there is a large degree of uncertainty for both the surgeon and the family. To help in decision making, it is important to have as much information about the kidney as possible. In looking at the progress of a kidney, it is important not to forget the antenatal ultrasound as a source of information. Many children can be managed conservatively, but they need close and prolonged follow-up if the hydronephrosis persists.

Suggested reading

Ransley P, Dhillon H, Gordon I, et al. The postnatal management of hydronephrosis diagnosed by prenatal ultrasound. *J Urol.* 1994;144:584–7.

Dhillon H. Prenatally diagnosed hydronephrosis: the Great Ormond Street experience. *Br J Urol.* 1998;81(suppl 2):39–44.

9 | Congenital Anomalies of the Bladder and Urethra

Mohan S. Gundeti and Imran Mushtaq

CASE 1

A 3-day-old male neonate is referred to your unit with an antenatal history of bilateral hydronephrosis. He has reportedly passed urine with a good stream but has a palpable bladder. His serum creatinine is 105 μmol/l. A renal ultrasound scan and micturating cystogram have been performed and are shown below.

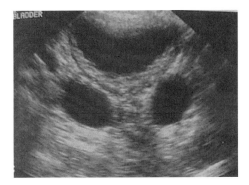

Fig. 9.1 Renal ultrasound.

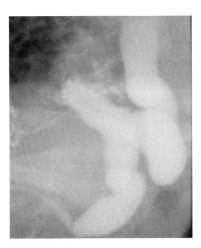

Fig. 9.2 Micturating cystogram.

1 What is the differential diagnosis in a male neonate with antenatal bilateral hydronephrosis?
2 What features are shown in Fig.9.1?
3 What abnormalities are seen in Fig. 9.2?
4 What is your initial management of this patient?
5 Which factors in this child's antenatal history and postnatal investigations are relevant in determining his prognosis?

Discussion

1 Any male neonate with prenatally detected bilateral hydronephrosis must be considered to have posterior urethral valves until investigations prove otherwise. Other more rare causes of infravesical obstruction include syringocele, urethral hypoplasia, and anterior urethral valves. Other conditions that may present with bilateral hydronephrosis include pelvi-ureteric junction obstruction, duplex kidneys, vesicoureteric reflux, and vesicoureteric junction obstruction.
2 The ultrasound image shows a thick-walled bladder with dilated ureters behind the bladder.
3 The cystogram shows a dilated posterior urethra, a prominent bladder neck, bladder diverticula, and vesicoureteric reflux. All these features are classical of posterior urethral valves.
4 Immediate decompression of the bladder with a urethral or suprapubic catheter for drainage is essential. Monitor serum electrolytes, creatinine, and acid-base balance daily until these parameters stabilize. Careful management of the fluid balance is mandatory as there will be a period of diuresis following catheterization. The involvement of a pediatric nephrologist at an early stage in the child's management is highly recommended. Once the renal function and electrolytes stabilize, the child will need to undergo ablation (resection, fulguration) of the valves. It is becoming increasingly popular to perform circumcision at the same time as valve ablation to reduce the risk of urinary tract infection.
5 Oligohydramnios, early prenatal detection (<24 weeks gestation), and high β-2 macroglobulin levels are poor antenatal prognostic factors. In the postnatal period, bilateral vesicoureteric reflux and a nadir creatinine greater than 70 μmol/l are associated with a poor renal outcome. Urinoma formation, bladder diverticula, urinary ascites, and reflux into a nonfunctioning kidney are pressure-relieving mechanisms associated with a better renal prognosis and improved bladder function.

Suggested reading

Ghanem MA. Long term bladder dysfunction and renal function in boys with posterior urethral valves based on urodynamic findings. *J Urol.* 2004;171(6 pt 1): 2409–12.

Jaureguizar E. The valve bladder: etiology and outcome. *Curr Urol Rep.* 2002;3(2):115–20.

Karmarkar SJ. Long-term results of surgery for posterior urethral valves: a review. *Pediatr Surg Int.* 2001;17(1):8–10.

Lopez Pereira P. Posterior urethral valves: prognostic factors. *BJU Int.* 2003;91(7):687–90.

Pinette MG. Enlarged fetal bladder: differential diagnosis and outcomes *J Clin Ultrasound.* 2003;31(6):328–34.

Podesta M. Bladder function associated with posterior urethral valves after primary valve ablation or proximal urinary diversion in children and adolescents. *J Urol.* 2002;168(4 pt 2):1830–5; discussion 1835.

CASE 2

A 2-week-old male neonate is referred for the investigation of prenatally detected bilateral hydronephrosis. Ultrasound examination of the urinary tract shows mild bilateral hydronephrosis and a non–thick-walled bladder. A routine micturating cystogram is performed and is shown below (Fig. 9.3).

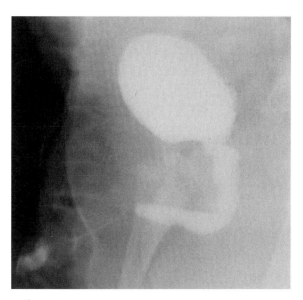

Fig. 9.3 Micturating cystogram.

1 Describe the findings seen in Fig. 9.3.
2 What is the most likely diagnosis?

3 What is the embryological origin of this abnormality?
4 What can be the presenting features?
5 How can the diagnosis be made?
6 What treatment may be required?

Discussion

1 The cystogram shows a dilated posterior and bulbar urethra. The anterior urethra is of a relatively small caliber in comparison.
2 The most likely diagnosis in this case is a syringocele.
3 Cowper's glands (bulbourethral glands) are situated in the urogenital diaphragm and along the corpous spongiosum of the bulbomembranous and bulbospongiosus urethra. Dilatation of these glands is described as a syringocele.
4 A syringocele can cause infravesical obstruction in males, which may cause hydronephrosis in the antenatal period. More often, however, syringoceles are asymptomatic and diagnosed incidentally during investigation for nonspecific symptoms such as dribbling, urgency, and hematuria.
5 The diagnosis can be made by a MCUG and confirmed endoscopically.
6 Most often, spontaneous perforation or rupture as a consequence of instrumentation does not require further treatment. If obstruction persists, transurethral incision is recommended. Occasionally, open surgical correction with marsupialization is required for very large syringoceles. Follow-up cystogram is useful to evaluate the urethra after surgical intervention.

Suggested reading

Bevers RF. Cowper's syringocele: symptoms, classification and treatment of an unappreciated problem. *J Urol.* 2000;163(3):782–4.

Dewan PA. A study of the relationship between syringoceles and Cobb's collar. *Eur Urol.* 1996;30(1):119–24.

Maizels M. Cowper's syringocele: a classification of dilatations of Cowper's gland duct based upon clinical characteristics of 8 boys. *J Urol.* 1983; 129(1):111–14.

Turker Koksal I. Unexpected presentation of syringocele. Acontractile bladder. *Urol Int.* 2003;71(2):222–3.

CASE 3

A 2-month-old male infant is referred by his general practitioner because his parents have noticed clear fluid coming from the anus at nappy changes.

His nappies are normally wet, and the parents report seeing drops of urine from the external urethral meatus. Your examination reveals a normal penis but an anteriorly placed anus. Micturating cystogram reveals the following findings (shown below):

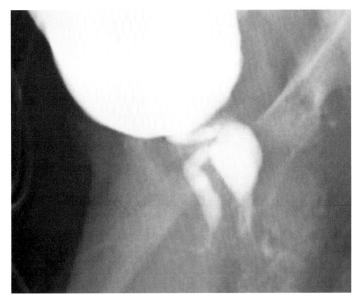

Fig. 9.4 Micturating cystogram.

1 What is shown in the cystogram, and what is the most likely diagnosis?
2 How are abnormalities of this type is classified?
3 What investigation would you like to perform to confirm the diagnosis?
4 What are the surgical options?
5 What advice would you give the parents regarding future continence?

Discussion

1 The cystogram shows a stenotic orthotopic urethra and a larger caliber ventral urethra opening into the perineum. This type of abnormality of the urethra is known as Y-type urethral duplication, congenital urethroperineal fistula, or congenital H-type urethroanal fistula. Mainly reported in young children, it is sometimes discovered only in adulthood. This abnormality is due to a failure in the alignment of the urethral folds of Tourneux and Rathke, so that a congenital urethroperineal fistula is formed.

2 The classification described by Effmann, Lebowitz, and Colodny is the most commonly used:

Type 1: Blind incomplete urethral duplication or accessory urethra.

  1A Distal: opens on the dorsal or ventral surface of the penis but does not communicate with the urethra or bladder.

  1B Proximal: blind ending channel arising from the urethra.

Type 2: Complete patent urethral duplication.

  2A Two meati.

   2A1: Two noncommunicating urethras independently arising from the bladder.

   2A2: Second channel arises from the first and courses independently into a second meatus.

  2B One meatus.

   2B1: The urethra splits into two and then reunites.

Type 3: Urethral duplication as a component of partial or complete caudal duplication.

3 An antegrade voiding cystourethrogram via a suprapubic tube is the most helpful investigation to delineate the anatomy of the urethra. In cases of incomplete visualization of both channels, a retrograde urethrogram, cystourethroscopy, and, on occasions, suprapubic cystoscopy are helpful in defining the anatomy. The information obtained is helpful in planning surgical reconstruction. Renal ultrasound, spinal ultrasound, and spinal X-ray are recommended in all cases because of the strong association with renal, vertebral, and sacral anomalies.

4 There are two surgical options: sequential dilatation of the orthotopic urethra (PADUA procedure) and a staged reconstruction approach. The latter approach involves mobilizing the ventral functional urethra to form a perineal urethrostomy, followed by a two-stage repair of the resulting perineal hypospadias.

5 The parents need to be counseled about the risk of urinary incontinence that can be a consequence of damage to the external sphincter during surgical reconstruction or may be due to an associated neuropathic bladder. The parents should also be warned about the risk of fecal incontinence in cases where an anorectal anomaly is also present.

Suggested reading

Ortolano V, Nasrallah PF. Urethral duplication. *J Urol.* 1986;136:909–12.

Podesta ML. Urethral duplication in children: surgical treatment and results. *J Urol.* 1998 Nov;160(5):1830–3.

Wagner JR. Congenital posterior urethral perineal fistulae: a unique form of urethral duplication. *Urology.* 1996;48(2):277–80.

Woodhouse CR. Duplication of the lower urinary tract in children. *BJU Int.* 1979;51:481–7.

CASE 4

A 9-year-old boy is referred by his general practitioner with a 5-week history of blood staining of his underwear. There is no history of hematuria, dysuria, or frequency of micturition. Midstream urine culture failed to reveal evidence of a urinary tract infection. Ultrasound of the renal tract shows two normal kidneys, a normal bladder that empties to completion, and no renal tract calculi. At cystoscopy the abnormality shown in Fig. 9.5 is seen in the bulbar urethra.

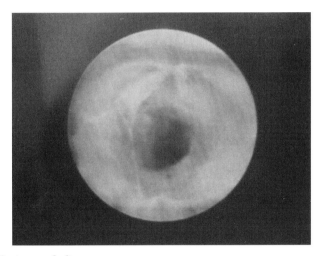

Fig. 9.5 Cystoscopy findings.

1 Describe the appearances seen in this urethra.
2 What is the name given to this condition, and why does it occur?
3 What other investigation would you consider in this patient?
4 What advice would you give to his parents?

Discussion

1 The urethra shows signs of inflammation, with areas of leukoplakia and fibrinous membrane covering these areas.
2 The history and cystoscopic findings are characteristic of urethritis posterior (also known as urethrorrhagia idiopathica). It occurs typically in prepubertal and pubertal boys, who complain of drops of blood appearing

at the end of micturition. Dysuria is a common feature, but gross hematuria is unusual. Bleeding occurs from an area of intense inflammation in the bulbar urethra just distal to the external sphincter. The etiology is unknown, although the onset just before or during puberty would suggest that endocrine factors might play a role.

3 As the history and cystoscopic findings are so characteristic, a biopsy of the affected area is not necessary. Histological findings include squamous metaplasia and epithelial hyperplasia. Microscopic examination of the urine with microbiological culture should always be performed to further confirm the diagnosis and exclude infection. A renal tract ultrasound is mandatory to exclude other pathologies, while a micturating cystogram is unlikely to reveal a detectable abnormality.

4 The parents and child should be reassured that urethritis posterior is a benign and self-limiting condition. Repeated cystoscopic examination is unhelpful and should be avoided.

Suggested reading

Docimo SG. Idiopathic anterior urethritis in prepubertal and pubertal boys: pathology and clues to etiology. *Urology*. 1998;51(1):99–102.

Dewan PA, Wilson TM. Idiopathic urethritis in the adolescent male. *Eur Urol*. 1996;30(4):494–7.

Harrison SC. Idiopathic urethritis in male children. *Br J Urol*. 1987;59(3):258–60.

Van Howe RS. Aetiology of idiopathic anterior urethritis. *Urology*. 1999;53(3):658.

CASE 5

A 2-year-old boy is referred with a history of recurrent urinary tract infections. An ultrasound scan shows left hydroureteronephrosis. A micturating cystogram is performed, and the findings are shown in Fig. 9.6.

1 Describe the findings of the cystogram.

2 What is the etiology of this abnormality?

3 What are the associated abnormalities?

4 What are the indications for surgical management?

Discussion

1 The micturating cystogram shows left vesicoureteral reflux with a paraureteral diverticulum (also called congenital bladder diverticulum). The urethra appears normal.

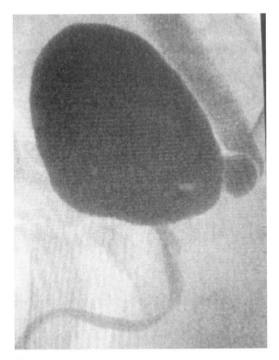

Fig. 9.6 Micturating cystogram.

2 The diverticulum seen in this patient has all the characteristic features of a congenital bladder diverticulum. It is solitary, occurs in a smooth-walled bladder, and is located adjacent to the lateral cornu of the trigone. An inherent weakness in the detrusor musculature is believed to be the etiology. Congenital diverticula are seen in association with Menkes' syndrome, Ehlers-Danlos syndrome, and prune-belly syndrome.

Acquired bladder diverticula are usually multiple and associated with a trabeculated bladder. They are usually the result of bladder outlet obstruction (posterior urethral valves, urethral stricture, neuropathic bladder dysfunction, and detrusor sphincter dyssynergia) infection or are iatrogenic.

3 Vesicoureteric reflux is commonly seen in association with such diverticula. The two entities may simply coexist or the diverticulum may have a causal relationship with vesicoureteric reflux, particularly in cases where the ureteric orifice becomes incorporated into the diverticulum on bladder filling. Reflux seen in such cases may resolve spontaneously, although in boys the likelihood of resolution is considered to be less than in girls. In a small number of cases, diverticula may cause ureteric obstruction and ipsilateral renal dysplasia.

4 The indications for surgical intervention include recurrent urinary tract infection, ureteric obstruction, or bladder outlet obstruction. Surgical options include diverticulectomy alone (bladder outlet obstruction), diverticulectomy with ureteric reimplantation (vesicoureteric reflux), or diverticulectomy with nephroureterectomy (renal dysplasia).

Suggested reading

Jayanthi VR. Extravesical detusorrhapy for refluxing ureters associated with parauretaral diverticula. *Urology.* 1995;45:664.

Leveard G. Urinary bladder diverticula and the Ehlers-Danlos syndrome in children. *J Paediatr Surg.* 1989;24:1184.

Livne PM. Congenital bladder diverticula causing ureteral obstruction *Urology.* 1985;25:273.

Pieretti RV. Congenital bladder diverticula in children. *J Paediatr Surg.* 1999;34:468.

Sarihan H. Congenital bladder diverticula in infants. *Eur Urol.* 1998;33:101.

10 | Genitourinary Trauma

Gerald Mingin, Peter D. Furness III,
and Martin A. Koyle

CASE 1

A 10-year-old boy is referred by his family practitioner for evaluation of a persistent, painless erection of 7 days' duration. There is no report of direct perineal trauma. However, the patient did fall while riding his bicycle just prior to the onset of symptoms.

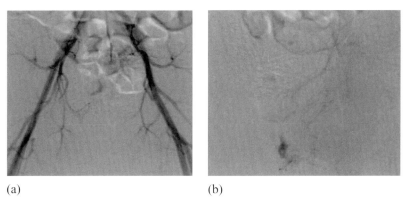

(a)   (b)

Fig. 10.1 (a) Arteriogram of the femoral and internal pudendal arteries. (b) Characteristic blush of the arterovenous fistula.

1 What is this boy's most likely diagnosis, and what is the etiology of this condition?
2 What diagnostic studies should be performed?
3 What is the current treatment for this condition?
4 What information would you relate to the patient and his family regarding prognosis?

Discussion

1 The most likely diagnosis is high-flow priapism. High-flow priapism is secondary to a traumatic arteriocavernous fistula seen in the setting of blunt perineal trauma. It is important to differentiate high-flow priapism from low-flow priapism, as the treatment is different in each case. Low-flow priapism is due to venous outflow obstruction leading to an engorgement of the corpora cavernosa. The factors causative for outflow obstruction include sickle cell anemia, leukemia, and any type of hypercoagulable state. Low-flow priapism is treated with corporeal irrigation after injection of a solution of 1:100,000 epinephrine. Persistent erection may require the creation of a corporeal spongiosal shunt. The fact that this patient does not have pain, in addition to likely sustaining a perineal injury, points to the diagnosis of high-flow priapism.

2 The patient should first undergo corporeal aspiration for blood gas analysis. If there is an elevation in oxygen saturation, the next step is Doppler ultrasonography. If on ultrasound the findings are suggestive of increased systolic velocity in the cavernosal arteries, standard or magnetic resonance imaging (MRI) angiography will confirm the diagnosis.

3 If spontaneous resolution does not occur, selective embolization of the fistula may be considered. This is performed by cannulating the femoral artery and accessing the fistula via the internal pudendal artery. Gel foam or platinum coils may be used for the embolization.

4 Although relatively new, the success rate of embolization appears high. In the literature, seven out of seven patients treated with embolization had resolution of their priapism. Only one patient required repeat embolization. Delayed detumescense was reported in 50% of these patients, with eventual complete resolution. In addition, normal erection was noted in all of the patients on follow-up.

Suggested reading

Eracleous E, Kondou M, Aristidou K, et al. Use of doppler ultrasound and 3-dimensional contrast-enhanced MR angiography in the diagnosis and follow-up of post-traumatic high flow priapism in a child. *Ped Rad.* 2000;30:265–7.

Shankar KR, Babar S, Rowlands P, Jones MO. Posttraumatic high flow priapism: treated with selective embolisation. *Ped Surg Int.* 2000;16:454–6.

Volkmer BG, Nesslauer T, Kraemer SC, Goerich J, Basche S, Gottfried HW. Prepubertal high flow priapism: incidence, diagnosis and treatment. *J Urol.* 2001;166:1018–22.

CASE 2

A 10-year-old boy is evaluated in the emergency department after sustaining a severe pelvic crush injury in a motor vehicle accident. The patient's vital signs are stable, and his physical examination reveals marked suprapubic tenderness and blood at the urethral meatus after partial void.

1 What studies would constitute an appropriate urologic workup in this patient?

2 What would be the most likely findings to explain his bleeding?

3 What course of treatment would you recommend?

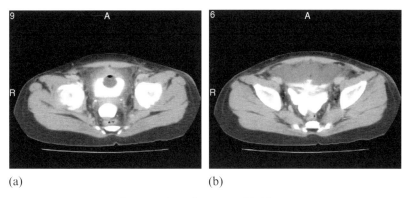

(a)   (b)

Fig. 10.2 Extravasation of contrast from the urinary bladder.

Discussion

1 After appropriate trauma resuscitation and stabilization of this patient, urologic evaluation starts with a review of the pelvic bony structures. Radiographic examination should include a pelvic anterior and posterior scout film, since pelvic fractures significantly increase the suspicion of a concomitant urethral or bladder injury. The next diagnostic studies to be performed are the standard urethrogram and cystogram to evaluate both the urethra and bladder. The urethrogram should be done first to be assured of urethral integrity prior to placing the catheter into the bladder. Never place a catheter across the urethra in the presence of blood at the meatus; doing so may convert a partial urethral disruption into a complete disruption. If the patient requires computer tomographic (CT) imaging for the evaluation of concomitant injuries, a CT cystogram may suffice to evaluate the bladder and not the urethra. The bladder must be filled to capacity with contrast from the study or by instillation, and postdrainage CT films must be obtained to rule out bladder rupture accurately.

2 The most likely finding would be a bladder rupture with or without a possible urethral injury. Clinically, gross hematuria is usually seen with bladder rupture; associated findings include suprapubic tenderness and inability to void. Urethral injury is frequently associated with blood per meatus in the absence of voiding as well as the butterfly perineal bruise, which this patient did not have. Bladder rupture as well as posterior urethral injury, is associated with a pelvic fracture sustained during a motor vehicle accident. Bladder rupture can be classified as either intraperitoneal or extraperitoneal. Intraperitoneal rupture is more common in young children where the bladder is intra-abdominally positioned. Intraperitoneal rupture occurs when the bladder sustains a sudden increase in pressure, leading to rupture of the bladder dome. With rupture of the overlying peritoneum, urine will extravasate into the peritoneal cavity.

3 Treatment for an intraperitoneal or extraperitoneal rupture associated with an embedded fragment of bone is open surgical debrediment and repair, with or without placement of a suprapubic catheter. Extraperitoneal rupture may be treated solely with catheter drainage for a period of 2–3 weeks. In either case, a cystogram is performed at the time of catheter removal to ensure complete healing.

Suggested reading

Iverson AJ, Morey AF. Radiographic evaluation of suspected bladder rupture following blunt trauma: critical review. *World J Surg.* 2001;25:1588–91.

Tarman GJ, Kaplan GW, Lerman SL, McAleer IM, Losasso BE. Lower genitourinary and pelvic fractures in pediatric patients. *Urology.* 2002;59(1):123–126.

CASE 3

A 15-year-old boy is referred by his family practitioner for right scrotal pain and nausea after being tackled in a soccer match the previous day.

1 What is the differential diagnosis?
2 What is the best diagnostic test to perform?
3 How would you manage this child?

Discussion

1 The most likely diagnosis would include testicular contusion, rupture, or dislocation. However, even in the presence of a traumatic etiology, the differential would also include testicular torsion, torsion of the appendix testis, and epididymitis. Any of these conditions may present with severe scrotal pain and tenderness, nausea, emesis, and urinary retention. Clinically, the scrotum may be tense, edematous, and ecchymotic. Blunt injuries to the testes account for the majority of testicular injuries. Because of the mobility of the testicle, these injuries are rare. However, the testicle can be compressed against the pubic bone, leading to contusion or rupture.

2 The most useful diagnostic tool in the evaluation of closed testicular trauma is ultrasonography of the scrotum. Intratesticular areas of sonolucency, as well as hyperechoic and hypoechoic regions with poorly defined testicular margins, are suggestive of testicular rupture or hematoma.

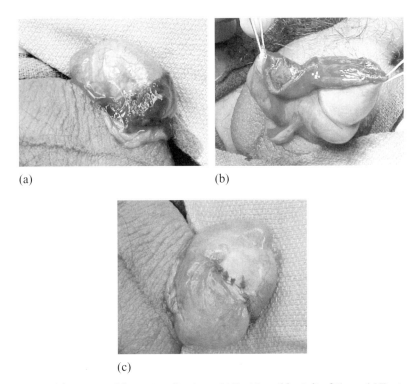

(a)   (b)

(c)

Fig. 10.3 (a) Rupture of the tunica albuginea. (b) Excision of devitalized tissue. (c) Tunica albuginea brought together.

3 If rupture of the testicle is suspected, the treatment is scrotal exploration with debridement of devitalized tissue and closure of the tunica albuginea (Fig. 10.3).

Suggested reading

Corrales JG, Corbel L, Cipolla B, Staerman F, Darnault P, Guille F. Accuracy of ultrasound diagnosis after blunt testicular trauma. *J Urol.* 1993;150(6):1834–6.

Ko SF, Ng SH, Wan YL, et al. Testicular dislocation: an uncommon and easily overlooked complication of blunt abdominal trauma. *Ann Emerg Med.* 2004;43(3):371–5.

Micallef M, Ahmad I, Ramesh N, Hurley M, McInerney D. Ultrasound features of blunt testicular injury. *Injury.* 2001;32(1):23–6.

CASE 4

A 13-year-old boy presents to the emergency department with bright red blood at the urethral meatus and an inability to void after having landed inappropriately on a pogo stick 6 hours prior to admission. The Clinical appearance of the perineum and findings of a retrograde urethrogram are shown in Figs. 10.4 and 10.5 respectively.

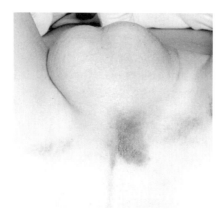

Fig. 10.4

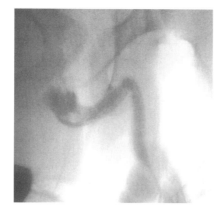

Fig. 10.5

1 What is the most likely diagnosis?
2 What imaging modality should be performed?
3 What constitutes the most appropriate treatment?

Discussion

1 The most likely diagnosis is a bulbar urethral injury. The hematoma is contained within Colles's fascia.
2 Provided that this is an isolated perineal injury and that the child has no associated injuries, a retrograde urethrogram would be the diagnostic

test of choice. If the patient had no blood at the urethral meatus, it would have been acceptable to attempt placement of a urethral catheter. In this case the patient has evidence of extravasation of contrast at the level of the bulbar urethra with no passage into the membranous urethra, suggestive of urethral transection.

3 The course of treatment is based on the preference of the surgeon. Urethral injury is a much more controversial topic, and for the interested reader the references have been provided below. The possible options for treatment include primary urethral repair, placement of a suprapubic tube with delayed repair, and endoscopic primary realignment. If an incomplete or complete injury is identified, then suprapubic tube urinary diversion is the time-tested standard of care. Follow-up urethrogram at 1 month with a subsequent suprapubic tube clamping schedule can be performed as long as the urethra has healed adequately. If the urethrogram and voiding are satisfactory, a uroflow with postvoid residual should be performed in 3–4 months to look for a delayed scar. If the urethrogram shows a significant scar or obstruction, a formal open urethroplasty should be planned at 3–6 months out from the injury. Primary urethral realignment in the pediatric urologic practice has not been widely accepted. Endoscopic therapy can be attempted with gentle passage of a guidewire across the defect provided that the urethra is not completely transected. Although a urethral stricture is still likely, the patient may be spared open surgery. In addition, primary realignment at the time of injury is acceptable in the case of an anterior urethral transection; however, this not the case with posterior injuries, where primary repair in the presence of a large hematoma may lead to urinary incontinence.

Suggested reading

Flynn B, Delvecchio FC, Webster GD. Perineal repair of pelvic fracture urethral distraction defects: 120 patients during the last 10 years. *J Urol.* 2003;170:1877–80.

Morey AF, McAninch JW. Reconstruction of posterior urethral disruption injuries: outcome analysis in 82 patients. *J Urol.* 1997;157(2):506–10.

Podesta ML, Jordan GH. Pelvic fracture urethral injuries in girls. *J Urol.* 2001;165:1660–5.

CASE 5

An 8-year-old previously healthy female falls forward over the handlebars of her bicycle. On evaluation, she is in moderate discomfort with stable vital signs and has a periumbilical hematoma. Her hematocrit is normal, but

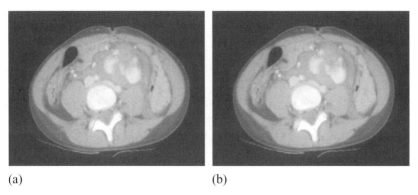

(a)   (b)

Fig. 10.6 Films demonstrating hematoma formation around a pelvic kidney.

urinalysis of a clear urine specimen is strongly dip positive for blood and there are more than 50 red blood cells per high-power field (RBC/HPF).

1 What is the most appropriate step in the evaluation and management of this patient?

2 What is the entity that is demonstrated in the images below?

3 What are the long-term recommendations in a patient such as this?

Discussion

1 Although hematuria is not an ideal indicator of renal injury, less than 2% of all major renal injuries in children will present with insignificant hematuria (<50 RBC/HPF). The abdominal CT, rather than intravenous urography, has become the imaging study of choice in the evaluation of abdominal trauma. Not only does it reveal superior anatomical detail, allowing one to grade the degree of renal trauma, but it also allows evaluation of other intra-abdominal organs.

2 This patient has a preexisting condition and a solitary pelvic kidney and has sustained a relatively minor blunt (grade 2) injury associated with a perirenal hematoma (Fig. 10.6). In children, it has been shown that congenitally abnormal kidneys are much more susceptible to injury, even from minor traumatic events.

3 Initially, this child will be only observed, without plans for further imaging. Abscess and delayed bleeding are potential subacute sequelae, although unlikely with this degree of renal injury. Rarely, in the long run, hypertension is seen, mediated by the rennin-angiotensin system or because of compression causing the "page kidney." Thus, periodic blood pressure monitoring is recommended. It is controversial as to what limits should be placed on individuals with known renal anomalies who wish to participate in contact sports. Appropriate counseling is mandatory in this group.

Suggested reading

Brown SL, Elder JS, Spirnak JP. Are pediatric patients more susceptible to major renal injury from blunt trauma? A comparative study. *J Urol.* 1998;161:138.

Levy JB, Baskin LS, Ewalt D, et al. Nonoperative management of blunt pediatric major renal trauma. *Urology.* 1993;42:423.

Morey AF, McAninch JW. Efficacy of radiographic imaging in pediatric blunt renal trauma. *J Urol.* 1996;156:2014.

Stein JP, Kaji DM, Eastman J, et al. Blunt renal trauma in the pediatric population: indications for radiological evaluation. *Urology.* 1994;44:409.

11 | Office Pediatric Urology

Ewen MacKinnon and Prasad Godbole

CASE 1

A 3-year-old boy is referred by his family practitioner for your opinion regarding a circumcision. He has a 6-month history of ballooning of his foreskin on micturition and two episodes of inflammation of the tip of his prepuce that resolved spontaneously. The appearances of the foreskin are shown below (Fig. 11.1a).

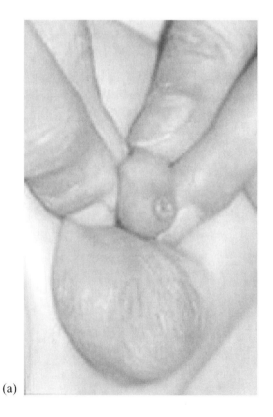

(a)

Fig. 11.1

1 How would you describe the foreskin?
2 What is the natural history of the foreskin depicted above?

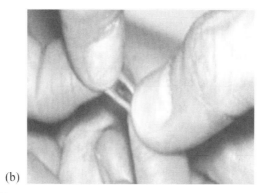

(b)

Fig. 11.1 (Contd.)

3 Would you perform a circumcision?
4 What advice would you give the parents?
5 What are your indications for circumcision?

Discussion

1 The foreskin can be best described as a healthy nonretractile foreskin. On gentle retraction, the inner layer of the prepuce "pouts" as opposed to the rigid noncompliant prepuce of balanitis xerotica obliterans (BXO). Spence in 1964 described how on drawing it forward by grasping the margins (Fig. 11.1b) an adequate lumen to the foreskin can be demonstrated for the purposes of micturition. The term *phimosis*, although used to describe a nonretractile foreskin, should be reserved for a nonretractile foreskin secondary to pathological conditions such as BXO.

2 Most boys have a foreskin that is nonretractile at birth as a result of congenital prepucial adhesions. These separate spontaneously, and the foreskin becomes retractile in most cases by 5–7 years of age but up to 15 years of age.

3 A healthy but as yet nonretractile foreskin and ballooning of the foreskin on micturition is normal and *not* an indication for circumcision. In this case no surgical intervention is required.

4 The parents should be reassured and explained the natural history of the foreskin. They should be advised against forcible retraction of the foreskin. During episodes of inflammation a warm bath is usually all that is required.

5 Routine neonatal circumcisions are common in the United States but not in the United Kingdom and the rest of Europe. The only nonmedical indication for circumcision is on religious or cultural grounds – the "ritual" circumcision. Medical reasons for circumcision include (i) BXO or other pathological conditions affecting the foreskin; (ii) recurrent, severe, and frequent attacks of balanoposthitis not responding to conservative management; and (iii) the aim to try and reduce the incidence of urinary infections in children with abnormal urinary tracts such as posterior urethral valves or gross vesicoureteric reflux (this is not accepted by all authorities).

Suggested reading

Brinton LA, Li JY, Rong SD, et al. Risk factors for penile cancer: results from a case-control study in China. *Int J Cancer*. Feb 1991;47(4):504–9.

Gairdner D. The fate of the foreskin. *BMJ*. 1949;2:1433–7.

Rickwood AM. Medical indications for circumcision. *BJU Int*. 1999;83(suppl 1):45–51.

Rickwood AM, Kenny SE, Donnell SC. Towards evidence based circumcision of English boys: survey of trends in practice. *BMJ*. 2000;321(7264):792–3.

Weiss C. Routine non-ritual circumcision in infancy. A new look at an old operation. *Clin Pediatr*. 1964;66:560–3.

CASE 2

A year later his mother, recently diagnosed with breast cancer, has found a swelling on the shaft of his penis (Fig. 11.2).

The swelling is soft though described by mother as being "firm," and she thinks there is a smaller one on the other side of the penis. At times it seems to be on the penile shaft, but on careful inspection it can be demonstrated to lie at the level of the coronal sulcus. It has an elliptical shape lying in a transverse plane. The mother is worried about cancer.

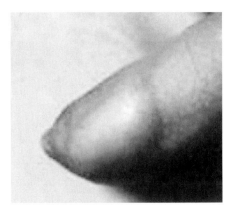

Fig. 11.2

1 What is this condition?
2 Can it be present with a retractable foreskin?

3 What is the natural history?
4 What should be done about it?
5 What other benign swelling is sometimes found at this level on the penis?

Discussion

1 The swelling is a plaque of smegma, which is a completely normal material created by desquamation of epithelial cells matted together with a small amount of mucous.
2 Smegma collects under the foreskin unless washed away. It can form whether or not the foreskin is retractable and can even form under the remains of foreskin after circumcision. It commonly is present while pre-pucial adhesions are present.
3 Smegma plaques spontaneously disappear. Sometimes they are seen emerging from the end of the foreskin, but often their disappearance is unnoticed.
4 Smegma does not cause inflammation. In fact so rarely, if ever, are pe-nile inflammatory conditions seen with retained smegma that it seems as though they provide a protective mechanism. They may have a bacterial protective effect in humans (in mature animals, this is not always so). The best course of action is to explain the situation to the parents and do noth-ing more. Forceful retraction of the foreskin in order to clean the plaque away causes distress to no good purpose. There is no validated evidence that it is carcinogenic.
5 Occasionally a child presents with a ventral midline inclusion dermoid of the prepuce. This too is benign and may be removed if the child or parents wish.

Suggested reading

Davenport M. ABC of general surgery in children;problems with the penis and prepuce. *BMJ*. 1996;312(7026):299–301.
Oster J. Further fate of the foreskin. Incidence of preputial adhesions, phimosis and smegma among Danish schoolboys. *Arch Dis Child*. 1968;43:200–203.

CASE 3

A 9-year-old boy presents to you with a 4-month history of dysuria, spraying on micturition, and occasionally bleeding from the foreskin on micturition. He is otherwise well. The appearances of the foreskin are shown below (Fig. 11.3).

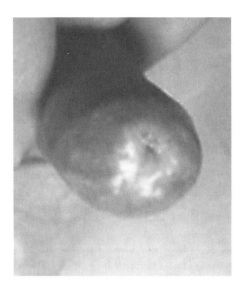

Fig. 11.3

1 What is your diagnosis?
2 What is the etiology and the pathology of the condition?
3 How would you manage this boy?
4 What are the long-term consequences of this condition?

Discussion

1 The appearances are typical of BXO. The foreskin is nonretractile and has a white sclerotic margin, which is rigid and noncompliant on attempted gentle retraction.

2 The etiology of BXO is unknown. It is considered to be the equivalent of lichen sclerosus in girls. It has been suggested that BXO may be due to inflammation with accentuation of the increased permeability of small blood vessels in a loose vascular region. Typically the inflammatory infiltrate is of lymphocytes. BXO is a chronic progressive inflammatory process in genital skin that in males results in sclerotic epithelial changes of the prepuce, glans penis, and urethral meatus individually or collectively. In adults it may ascend the urethra. The first cases described by Stuhmer and quoted by McKay et al. in 1928 were in circumcised adults. The later identification of the pathological process in the foreskin led some authors to suggest the term *posthitis xerotica obliterans*, but both the glans (*balanos*, "acorn": Greek) and foreskin (*posthos*, Greek) may be involved. It appears to have been much less common in children until recently, justifying a report of

4 cases in boys in 1975, while in adults it seems to predominate in an older age range. The incidence of BXO in boys presenting clinically is relatively low, though it seems to be on the increase, and the condition may often be missed or misdiagnosed. Rickwood et al. reported an incidence of 0.4 cases in 1000 boys per year or 0.6% of boys affected by their fifteenth birthday. Another study quotes the incidence as 9% in a review of 100 circumcisions performed for all reasons including culture. BXO may affect the glans in up to 20% of cases and the anterior urethra in a small minority. Recently there are increasing reports of the association of human papilloma virus with BXO, though a causal relationship has not been proven.

3 Classically, circumcision is the preferred treatment of choice to excise all the diseased mucosa of the foreskin. Topical steroid application to the prepucial ring to treat phimosis has reported success rates of between 33% and 95% in various series, but frequently authors fail to define clearly the difference between a nonretractile foreskin and a true BXO. Other nonsurgical methods have been described, including long-term antibiotic therapy, topical nonsteroidal cream, and sublesional injection of steroid, with variable results. Where clinically the condition is diagnosed but regarded as "mild," topical steroid creams have proved beneficial. For more established cases, foreskin meatoplasty and injection of triamcinolone are being evaluated with encouraging results (Godbole and MacKinnon, *unpublished observations*). In cases involving urethral meatus, meatal dilatation, meatotomy, or urethroplasty may be necessary.

4 BXO may affect the glans in children, but resolution usually occurs following treatment of the foreskin. Involvement of the anterior urethra occurs rarely in children. Progression of the disease process after circumcision may result in meatal stenosis. This resolution contrasts with the experience of adults, where a more chronic and progressive condition is seen. Untreated BXO in adults has been claimed to have a causal link with penile carcinoma.

Suggested reading

Aynaud O, Piron D, Casanova JM. Incidence of preputial lichen sclerosus in adults: histologic study of circumcision specimens. *J Am Acad Dermatol*. 1999;41(6):923–6.

Berdeu D, Sauze L, Ha-Vinh P, Blum-Boisgard C. Cost-effectiveness analysis of treatments for phimosis: a comparison of surgical and medicinal approaches and their economic effect. *BJU Int*. Feb. 2001;87(3):239–44.

Chalmers RJ, Burton PA, Bennett RF, et al. Lichen sclerosus et atrophicus. A common and distinctive cause of phimosis in boys. *Arch Dermatol*. 1984;120:1025–7.

McKay DL Jr, Fuqua F, Weinberg AG. Balanitis xerotica obliterans in children. *J Urol.* 1975;114(5):773–5.

Vincent MV, MacKinnon AE. The response of clinical BXO to the application of topical steroid based creams. *J Pediatr Surg.* In press.

CASE 4

A 6-month-old boy is referred with a history of extreme ballooning of his foreskin to the size of a golf ball and needing expression with every act of micturition (Fig. 11.4).

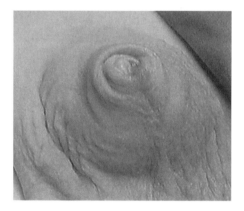

Fig. 11.4

1 What does this illustration show?

2 How should this be managed?

Discussion

1 This is known as mega-prepuce or "volcano penis." It is a condition of gross dilatation of the prepucial sac with an increase in connective tissue of the dartos layer. This seems to draw the mucosal surface downward until it envelopes the entire penile shaft. As a result the penis becomes buried. During micturition this sac distends enormously and buries the penis.

2 The dartos layer must be divided to release the penile shaft. Numerous techniques have been described for the same. The stretched foreskin can be resected, but there is a great danger of leaving the shaft covered by mucosal layer foreskin, which is not cosmetically satisfactory. Alternatively, a foreskin meatoplasty may be performed; this allows some regression of the condition. However, in most cases, redundant tissue needs excision at a later procedure. In this way the penile shaft can be covered with normal-looking shaft skin with a superior appearance.

Suggested reading

O'Brien A, Shapiro AM, Frank JD. Phimosis or congenital megaprepuce? *Br J Urol.* Jun 1994;73(6):719–20.

Powis MR, Capps S. Preputial intussusception or acquired megaprepuce. *Pediatr Surg Int.* Mar 1998;13(2–3):158–9.

Summerton DJ, McNally J, Denny AJ, Malone PS. Congenital megaprepuce: an emerging condition – how to recognize and treat it. *BJU Int.* Sep 2000;86(4):519–22.

CASE 5

A 15-year-old boy complaining of a dragging feeling in the left hemiscrotum is referred to you by his family doctor. The doctor has identified a varicocele and has requested advice as to whether surgery is needed.

1 What diagnostic classification is applied to varicoceles? Are they always primary lesions?

2 Is any intervention necessary? What are the options, and what are the indications for intervention in this patient?

3 If intervention is contemplated, what complications must be discussed with the patient and his family?

Discussion

1 A minimal degree of distension of the veins of the pampiniform plexus with the Valsalva maneuver is commonly seen in young adults. However, distinct dilatation under these circumstances with resolution at rest is grade 1, distension that is present on standing alone is grade 2, and prominent veins with symptoms of dragging discomfort is regarded as grade 3. Very rarely, there may be an intra-abdominal mass pressing on the gonadal vein causing obstruction. For this reason, some authorities recommend abdominal ultrasound examination in all cases. Others suggest that this is only advisable where there are unusual features, such as right-sided or bilateral lesions, or concomitant clinical features.

2 The prime indication for intervention is to alleviate symptoms of dragging discomfort that may be significant, as in this case. Impaired testicular growth may be caused by a varicocele, which is reversible following surgery. A varicocele may affect spermatogenesis, but studies are inconclusive regarding improving subfertility by treating a varicocele. The treatment option is either venous embolization or high division of the gonadal vessels (Palomo procedure), which may be accomplished laparo-scopically. In this operation, most surgeons divide the artery to the testis as well as the veins as vascularization is maintained from the artery to the vas and possibly from the gubernaculum. Occasionally, secondary veins draining away from the main gonadal vessels are present, and these need to be divided.

3 There is approximately a 10% chance of failure of the procedure either by embolization or surgery. There is also a 10% chance of hydrocele develop-ing even several years later.

Suggested reading

Diamond DA. Adolescent varicocele: emerging understanding. *BJU Int.* 2003;92(suppl 1):48–51.

Esposito C, Valla JS, Najmaldin A, et al. Incidence and management of hydrocele following varicocele surgery in children. *J Urol.* 2004;17:1271–3.

Fisch H, Hyun G, Hensle TW. Testicular growth and gonadotrophin response associated with varicocele repair in adolescent males. *BJU Int.* 2003;91:75–8.

Itoh K, Suzuki Y, Yazawa H, Ichiyanagi O, Miura M, Sasagawa I. Results and complications of laparoscopic Palomo varicocelectomy. *Arch Androl.* 2003;49(2):107–10.

Yeniyol CO, Tuna A, Yener H, Zeyrek N, Tilki A. High ligation to treat pain in varicocele. *Int Urol Nephrol.* 2003;35(1):65–8.

CASE 6

The mother of a 6-week-old boy has been referred to you because he has a swelling in the groin. The family doctor was not sure whether this was a femoral or inguinal hernia but said it had to be operated upon immediately for fear of incarceration. The infant was born at 32 weeks gestation and needed ventilation for 3 days.

1 Which type of hernia is this likely to be?
2 What advice would you give concerning the timing of surgery?
3 What warnings would you provide concerning complications from surgery?
4 Do inguinal herniae in infants ever disappear like hydroceles?

Discussion

1 Femoral herniae are uncommon in children and less common in boys than girls. These rarely present in the first few months of life. Virtually all inguinal herniae in children are of the indirect type.

2 There is a high risk of incarceration of an inguinal hernia in a child less than 6 months old, and so surgery must be planned as soon as possible. However, before the age of 52 weeks by gestational dates, and particularly in an infant who needed ventilation at birth, there is a significant risk of respiratory complications developing. Therefore the family need to be warned of the signs of incarceration of the hernia while awaiting surgery to be performed as soon as possible after the infant reaches 52 weeks gestational age.

3 In general, surgery for childhood herniae is very safe and has a low recurrence risk. However, although the overall recurrence in infancy is about 1%, in preterm infants the risk rises to about 5%. In such an infant there would be a chance of more than 75% that there is a contralateral patent processus vaginalis. On the other hand the risk of a hernia developing is only about 1:4 to 1:5. For this reason many surgeons recommend that the contralateral groin not be explored unless there are other features indicating it to be advisable.

The family must be also warned of the risk to the testis due to devascularization (about 10% in the preterm) or excision of a portion of the vas (about 0.33%). Retraction of the testis is also a rare complication. However, the risk to the testis from incarceration, particularly if operated upon as an emergency, is significantly greater than with elective surgery.

4 The processus vaginalis if not distended by fat or bowel may close spontaneously in the first 12 months of life. For this reason hydroceles may resolve, although in the presence of a CSF shunt or peritoneal dialysis they do not resolve. The processus vaginalis of a hernia does not close, though for a period of time herniation of omentum or bowel may cease and the hernia may seem to have resolved.

Suggested reading

Al-Shanafey S, Giacomantonio M. Femoral hernia in children. *J Pediatr Surg.* 1999; 34:1104–6.
Boley SJ, Cahn D, Lauer T, Weinberg G, Kleinhaus S. The irreducible ovary: a true emergency. *J Pediatr Surg.* 1991;26(9):1035–8.
Kumar VH, Clive J, Rosenkrantz TS, Bourque MD, Hussain N. Inguinal hernia in preterm infants. *Pediatr Surg Int.* 2002;18:147–52.
Misra D, Hewitt G, Potts SR, Brown S, Boston VE. Inguinal herniotomy in young infants, with emphasis on premature neonates. *J Pediatr Surg.* 1994;29:1496–8.
Surana R, Puri P. Is contralateral exploration necessary in infants with unilateral inguinal hernia? *J Pediatr Surg.* 1993;28:1026–7.

12 | Neuropathic Bladder and Bowel

Martin Kaefer

CASE 1

You are asked to evaluate a full-term newborn child for an abnormality involving the spine. The mother did not receive any perinatal care, nor did she undergo any prenatal screening. The appearance of the spine is shown below.

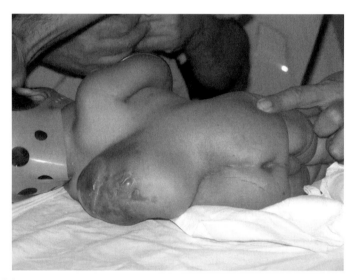

Fig. 12.1

1 What factors appear to be important in the etiology of this lesion? What preventative measures could have been taken by the mother that may have reduced the chance of developing this lesion in her newborn?
2 What are the implications of such a lesion for the urinary tract? What is the appropriate initial evaluation of this child from a urologic standpoint?
3 What abnormalities may be appreciated on renal ultrasound?
4 Does repair of the spinal cord defect affect bladder behavior?
5 What two primary purposes does the urodynamic evaluation serve?

Discussion

1 Myelodysplasia, defined as abnormal development of the vertebral column and spinal cord, is the most common etiology of neuropathic bladder dysfunction in children. A genetic component appears to be partially responsible for this disorder. In a family with one child with myelodysplasia, there exists a 2–5% chance that each subsequent sibling will suffer from the same condition. Early studies reported the incidence at 1 in 1000 live births. Dietary supplementation with folic acid (a metabolite important for proper spinal cord formation) can reduce the incidence of myelodysplasia by approximately 50%.

2 Incomplete closure and development of the spinal cord can result in disruption of the nerves responsible for (i) appropriate bladder accommodation to increasing volumes of urine and (ii) proper external urinary sphincter activity. Initial urologic evaluation of the child found to have spinal dysraphism should include a renal ultrasound and voiding cystourethrogram. In addition, random clean intermittent catheterization is performed on multiple occasions to determine if the child is retaining excess amounts of urine. If the volumes obtained during random catheterization are in excess of predicted capacity for age, then the parents are taught clean intermittent catheterization, which is to be performed after discharge to home.

3 As many as 15% of newborns will be found to have an abnormal upper urinary tract. The most common abnormality seen is hydronephrosis. Hydronephrosis is often secondary to abnormal lower urinary tract function and elevated intravesical pressures. A renal ultrasound serves the additional purpose of evaluating for renal fusion anomalies, which are more common in patients with myelodysplasia.

4 Repair of the spinal cord defect can, in a minority of cases, result in temporary spinal shock. The first urodynamic assessment is therefore typically delayed until after the child has reached at least 2 months of age.

5 Urodynamic evaluation serves two purposes. First, it serves as a baseline against which all future urodynamic evaluations can be compared. Changes in the urodynamic profile may be the first indication (often before lower extremity function changes) that postmyelomeningocele closure spinal cord tethering is occurring and that surgical intervention may be required. Second, it determines the overall storage characteristics of the bladder and sphincteric function. Three specific combinations of bladder contractility and external sphincter activity are seen: synergic voiding, dyssynergic voiding, and complete denervation.

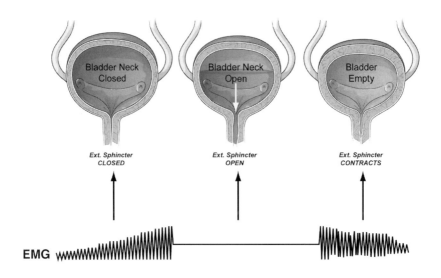

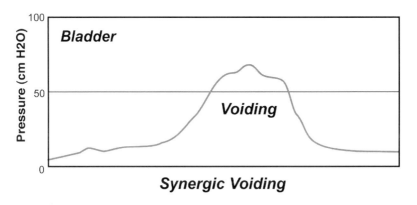

(a)

Fig. 12.2 (a) *Coordinated synergic voiding:* Electrical activity of the external urethral sphincter is chronically active. Just prior to experiencing a detrusor contraction the activity of the external sphincter is silenced, providing a marked decrease in urethral resistance and thereby facilitating emptying. Intravesical pressure is shown in the bottom panel (*Continued.*)

(Fig. 12.2) This system of classification is of great importance in predicting long-term renal and bladder function and thereby determining who will benefit from aggressive measures to minimize progressive urinary tract injury. Within the first 3 years of life, patients with a dyssynergic voiding pattern have a much higher incidence of urinary tract deterioration. There is mounting evidence that aggressively and proactively

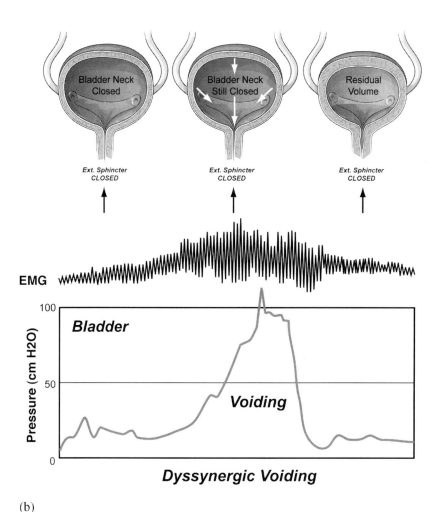

EMG

Pressure (cm H2O)

Bladder

Voiding

Dyssynergic Voiding

(b)

Fig. 12.2 (Contd.) (b) *Dyssynergic voiding:* In cases of neuropathic bladder dysfunction, dis-coordination between bladder and sphincter activity can often be appreciated. As the bladder begins to contract, the activity of the external sphincter actually increases, resulting in high outlet pressures and ineffective voiding. Intravesical pressure is shown in bottom panel. © IUSM, Office of Visual Media, with permission.

treating high-risk patients (those defined as having either high outlet re-sistance, detrusor sphincter dyssynergy, and/or bladder hypercontractil-ity, i.e. the so-called "hostile bladder dynamics") with clean intermittent catheterization and anticholinergic medications may substantially reduce the incidence of both upper urinary tract injury and long-term bladder dysfunction.

Suggested reading

Bauer S, Hallet M, Khoshbin S. The predictive value of urodynamic evaluation in the newborn with myelodysplasia. *JAMA*. 1984;152:650.

Edelstein RA, Bauer SB, Kelly MD, et al. The long-term urological response of neonates with myelodysplasia treated proactively with intermittent catheterization and anticholinergic therapy. *J Urol*. 1995;154(4):1500–4.

Hunt GM, Whitaker RH. The pattern of congenital renal anomalies associated with neural-tube defects. *Dev Med Child Neurol*. 1987;29(1):91–5.

Kaefer M, Pabby A, Kelly M, et al. Improved bladder function after prophylactic treatment of the high risk neurogenic bladder in newborns with myelomeningocele. *J Urol*. 1999;162(3 pt 2):1068–71.

Palomaki G, Williams J, Haddow J. Prenatal screening for open neural-tube defects in Maine. *N Engl J Med*. 1999;340:1049–50.

CASE 2

A 6-year-old child with a history of a closed myelomeningocele presents with a chief complaint of urinary incontinence. The child has not received any prior treatment for neuropathic bladder dysfunction. Ultrasound reveals severe bilateral hydronephrosis (not shown). The voiding cystourethrogram is shown in Fig. 12.3 (the child was unable to void at the end of this study).

1 What are the most likely causes for urinary incontinence in a child with myelomeningocele?

2 Does the level of the vertebral defect adequately predict the degree or level of neurologic impairment involving the bladder and sphincter?

3 A representation of this child's urodynamic study is shown in Fig. 12.4. The child did not leak at any time during the study. Describe the pressure tracing. Considering this urodynamic profile, is it surprising that the child has severe hydronephrosis and renal impairment?

4 High-pressure bladder dynamics often lead to renal injury. What is the first aspect of renal function to suffer in this situation? In light of this, what nonneurologic issue may be contributing to this child's incontinence and further urinary tract decompensation?

5 What medical means are there for treating this patient's incontinence?

Discussion

1 Both detrusor and sphincteric dysfunction must be considered when determining the etiology of urinary incontinence in a child with myelomeningocele. Detrusor instability can result in intravesical pressures that overcome sphincteric resistance even at low bladder volumes.

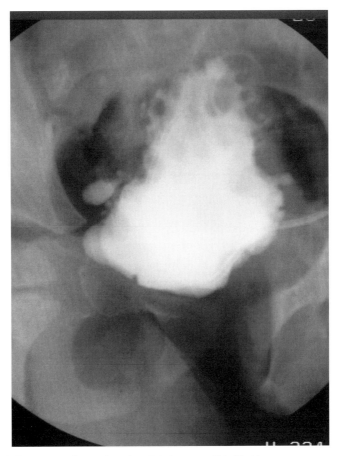

Fig. 12.3 Cystogram of severely trabeculated neuropathic bladder.

Sphincteric incompetence with low outlet resistance is another frequently encountered cause of incontinence. Finally, elevated outlet resistance may result in overflow incontinence. Elevated outlet resistance can be fixed, as in the case of sphincteric fibrosis, by complete denervation. Elevated outlet resistance can also result from detrusor sphincter dyssynergy.

2 The level of the vertebral defect often fails to adequately predict the level of neurologic impairment. There are several reasons for this. First, spinal cord lesions are usually incomplete. It is therefore possible to see great differences in bladder and sphincter function between two children with the same level of bony defect. Children with higher lesions (i.e. high lumbar or thoracic) can also have complete reconstitution of portions of the spinal cord below the defect. Finally, in many children there can be associated abnormalities of the spinal cord superior to the bony defect. It is therefore

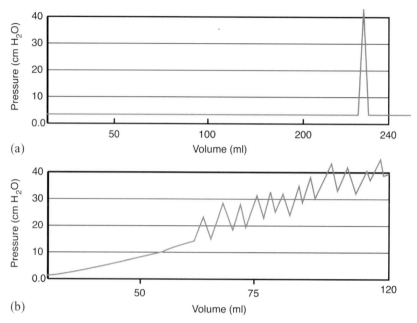

Fig. 12.4 (a) Urodynamic profile of a healthy child of age similar to the patient's. (b) Patient's urodynamic profile.

imperative that the child undergo formal urodynamic testing in order to establish the degree of lower urinary tract impairment.

3 The study demonstrates a hypertonic bladder with a steeply rising tonus limb, reflecting poor baseline bladder compliance. In addition, multiple high-amplitude uninhibited contractions are appreciated. The child did not leak during this study. It is therefore not surprising that renal injury has occurred. McGuire et al. were the first to demonstrate that patients with intravesical pressures in excess of $40 \, cm \, H_2O$ were significantly more likely to experience renal damage from a direct pressure effect and/or the presence of vesicoureteral reflux.

4 The first aspect of renal function to suffer in the presence of elevated intravesical pressures is concentrating ability. Poor concentrating ability in turn results in larger volumes of urine, which can overwhelm the existing storage capacity of the bladder. Establishing the volume of urine produced in a 24-hour period may help to explain the cause of the child's incontinence.

5 The key to successful treatment of this child's incontinence is providing a low-pressure environment for the storage of urine. Clean intermittent catheterization is used to provide timely evacuation of urine before a volume is reached at which elevated pressures are experienced. Anticholinergic medications serve to reduce bladder tonicity through a direct action on the muscarinic receptors. Use of sustained release formulations may result in reduced incidence of anticholinergic side effects and improved patient compliance. Recently, Koff et al. (2004) have advocated the use of a nighttime indwelling catheter to provide optimal bladder drainage. By improving nighttime drainage, they have documented significant improvement in hydronephrosis and bladder compliance.

Suggested reading

Bauer SB, Joseph DB. Management of the obstructed urinary tract associated with neurogenic bladder dysfunction. *Urol Clin N Am.* 1990;17(2):395–406.

Kaefer M, Bauer SB. The surgical correction of incontinence in myelodysplastic children. In: King L, ed. *Urologic Surgery in Infants and Children.* Philadelphia: Saunders; 1998.

Koff SA, Gigax MR, Jayanthi VR. Nocturnal bladder emptying: a simple technique for reversing urinary tract deterioration in children with neurogenic bladder [abstract]. Presented at the 2004 meeting of the American Academy of Pediatrics. Abstract 60.

McGuire EJ, Woodside JR, Borden TA, Weiss RM. Prognostic value of urodynamic testing in myelodysplastic patients. *J Urol.* 1981;126:205–9.

CASE 3

A 16-year-old athletic boy presents with a 6-month history of urinary and fecal incontinence. He has also noticed problems with balance while playing soccer. A picture of the boy's lumbosacral spine is shown in Fig. 12.5.

1 What are the important physical findings that can be appreciated on examination of this patient's lumbosacral spine?
2 What forms of radiographic and functional testing may be useful in determining if these physical findings are related to his incontinence?
3 From an embryologic perspective, how can one explain the occurrence of (i) a pigmented nevus and (ii) an intraspinal lipoma in this patient?
4 This boy was found to have an intraspinal lipoma. What is the mechanism for his incontinence?
5 In contrast to the cutaneous findings of a nevus, dimple, or hair patch, which are apparent at birth, why the physical finding of an asymmetric gluteal cleft (and urinary incontinence) might first become apparent only at a later age?

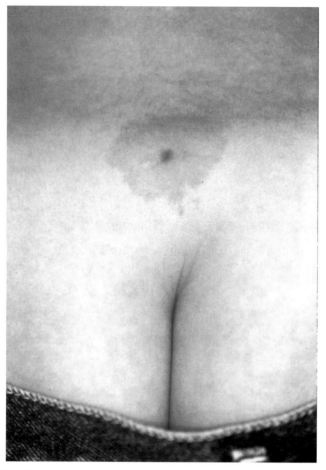

Fig. 12.5 Lumbosacral spine.

Discussion

1 There are three important physical findings demonstrated in this pho-
tograph: a sacral dimple, a pigmented nevus overlying the lumbosacral
spine, and an asymmetric gluteal cleft.
2 All patients with a cutaneous abnormality overlying the lower spine
should undergo a magnetic resonance imaging (MRI) of the lumbosacral
spine to evaluate for an intraspinal lesion. One of the most common lesions consists of an intraspinal lipoma that involves the spinal cord and
nerve roots. In the first 6 months of life, prior to ossification of the caudal
vertebral bones, it is also possible to evaluate for spinal cord tethering using a spinal ultrasound. Urodynamic testing will reveal abnormal lower

urinary tract function in about one third of babies with a tethering lesion and younger than 18 months of age. In contrast, practically all individuals older than 3 years of age who have not been operated on or in whom an occult dysraphism has been belatedly diagnosed have abnormal urodynamic profiles.

3 The spinal cord arises from the primitive ectoderm. In contrast, the surrounding soft tissue and bony structures develop from the primitive mesoderm. Aberrant neurulation (tubularization of the ectodermal layer into the neural tube) may result in an abnormal migration of these two primitive cell layers. As a result, other ectodermal elements (e.g. melanocytes and hair follicles) may be found in the dermis, leading to the presence of a pigmented nevus or a hair patch. In a similar fashion, mesodermal elements (e.g. lipocytes) may be found intertwined with neural elements of the spinal cord, resulting in a spinal cord lipoma.

4 Each of these physical findings is suggestive of an occult spinal abnormality, which can result in spinal cord tethering. Figure 12.6 demonstrates the normal relationships between the spinal cord and vertebra in the absence of a spinal cord lesion. The spinal column increases in axial length at a greater rate than does the spinal cord. As a result the spinal cord rises to a higher position. In contrast, with an intraspinal lipoma (shown in Fig. 12.6b), the spinal cord is fixed to a location along the vertebral column. As a result the spinal cord is unable to "float" upward and the cord is stretched. This stretching results in a relative state of hypoxia in the area of the distal cord and subsequent nerve injury to the distal spinal cord segments.

5 The neurologic effects and subsequent musculoskeletal implications of an occult spinal cord lipoma are often not appreciated until the child has undergone axial growth and the spinal cord has been put on stretch ("put on tether"). Once tethering has occurred, nerve injury is often not symmetric. As a result, growth and maintenance of the gluteal muscles on the more affected side are more significantly impaired. The more affected side undergoes significantly more atrophy. This results in a deviation of the gluteal crease to the more affected side (much like the deviation of the tongue to the side of a 12th cranial nerve injury).

Suggested reading

Bruce D, Schut L. Spinal lipomas in infancy and childhood. *Brain.* 1979;5:92.
Dick EA, Patel K, Owens CM, et al. Spinal ultrasound in infants. *BJR.* 2002;75(892):384.
Keating M, Rink R, Bauer S. Neuro-urologic implications of changing approach in management of occult spinal lesions. *J Urol.* 1988;140:1299.

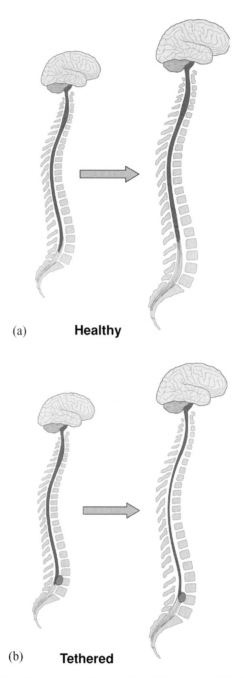

(a) **Healthy**

(b) **Tethered**

Fig. 12.6 (a) Position of normal spinal cord as the child matures. (b) Position of abnormal spinal cord anatomy with spinal cord Lipoma as the child matures.

CASE 4

A 10-year-old boy presents with a past history of low imperforate anus and new onset of constipation, urinary urgency, and urinary and fecal incontinence. Initial treatment for the imperforate anus consisted of a diverting colostomy and a subsequent rectal pull through operation at 18 months of age. Treatment with laxatives and anticholinergic medications has resulted in partial improvement of his symptoms.

1 Describe a possible nonneurogenic cause for this child's urinary urgency and urinary incontinence?

2 Describe a possible neurologic cause for the patient's symptoms.

3 What diagnostic evaluation should be undertaken in this setting?

4 What is the medical paradigm for treating fecal incontinence in a child with neuropathic bowel dysfunction secondary to spinal cord myelomeningocele or occult spinal cord tethering?

5 What surgical options are there for treating fecal incontinence if medical management fails?

Discussion

1 Constipation can contribute to bladder irritability from the mass effect on the posterior aspect of the bladder. In cases of severe constipation the stool bolus may also inhibit bladder emptying (Fig. 12.7). Poor bladder emptying has been shown to improve following treatment of constipation.

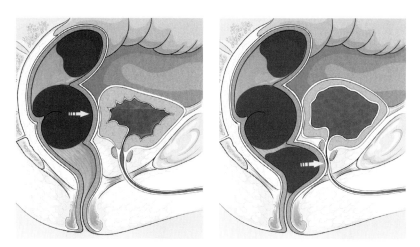

Fig. 12.7 The effect of constipation on bladder function. © IUSM, Office of Visual Media, with permission.

In one study, postvoid residual urine was shown to drop from 66% at baseline assessment to 21% following treatment of the constipation.

Stool in the rectum may push up on the posterior aspect of the bladder, resulting in bladder instability (left panel). Severe forms of constipation have the potential to externally compress the bladder neck and inhibit bladder emptying (right panel).

2 There is an increased incidence (up to 50%) of occult spinal cord abnormalities in individuals with anorectal malformations. Earlier reports demonstrated that the incidence varied proportionately in relation to the height of the rectal lesion, with spinal cord tethering more commonly seen in patients with high imperforate anus. However, one recent study suggests that the incidence may not differ significantly between patients with supralevator and infralevator lesions, underscoring the need to consider this diagnosis in all children with anorectal malformations.

3 All patients with an anorectal malformation should undergo an evaluation of the lumbosacral spinal cord. Although vertebral abnormalities are also commonly seen in patients with imperforate anus (VACTERL syndrome, i.e. V, vertebral; A, anorectal; C, cardiac; T, tracheal; E, esophageal; R, renal; L, limb), absence of a vertebral anomaly does not exclude the possibility of intraspinal pathology. MRI remains the most definitive method to evaluate for an intraspinal lesion. An alternative means for evaluating the lumbosacral spinal cord in the newborn setting is spinal ultrasound. This later method has the added advantage of not requiring a general anesthetic (i.e. a general anesthetic is often needed when performing MRI in the newborn in order to prevent movement artifact). Urodynamic evaluation should be undertaken if a spinal cord abnormality is noted.

4 Bowel function can improve after surgical release of spinal cord tethering. If complete improvement is not appreciated, then "controlled constipation" is the medical paradigm for treating fecal incontinence. Hard formed stool (which is less likely to pass across a weak, denervated anal sphincter) is allowed to accumulate and is released through the use of daily suppositories at an appropriate time.

5 In 1990, Malone described the concept of exploiting the flap valve principle to create a continent abdominal wall stoma through which an antegrade enema could be delivered. The Malone antegrade continence enema (MACE) (Fig. 12.8) has dramatically improved the quality of life of many individuals with neuropathic bowel dysfunction, allowing daily complete evacuation of the colon while one sits on the commode. Placement of a cecostomy tube or button, although a potentially less invasive means of creating access to the cecum, carries with it a higher chance of stomal leakage.

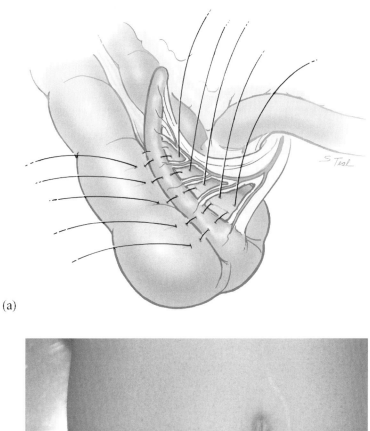

(a)

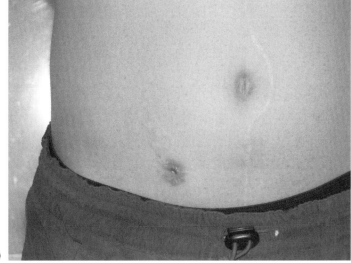

(b)

Fig. 12.8 (a) In situ MACE procedure: the appendix remains attached to the cecum and is folded into the tenea of the colon. Permanent sutures are used to bring neighboring cecal wall over the appendix and thereby create a flap valve. © IUSM of Visual Media, with permission. (b) MACE: abdominal wall stoma.

Suggested reading

Dohil R, Roberts E, Jones KV, et al. Constipation and reversible urinary tract abnormalities. *Arch Dis Child.* 1994;70(1):56–7.

Golonka NR, Haga LJ, Keating RP, et al. Routine MRI evaluation of low imperforate anus reveals unexpected high incidence of tethered spinal cord. *J Pediatr Surg.* 2002;37(7):966–9.

Malone PS, Ransley PG, Kiely EM. Preliminary report: the antegrade continence enema. *Lancet.* 1990;336(8725):1217–8.

Tsakayannis DE, Shamberger RC. Association of imperforate anus with occult spinal dysraphism. *J Pediatr Surg.* 1995;30(7):1010–12.

CASE 5

A 6-year-old boy presents with a chief complaint of recurrent urinary tract infections and urinary incontinence (Fig. 12.9).

1 Describe the findings shown in Fig. 12.9. Which radiographic imaging studies can be used to confirm the diagnosis?

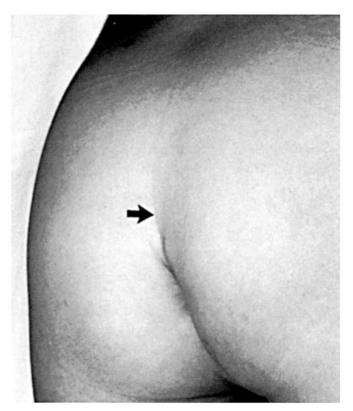

Fig. 12.9

2 Name the known risk factors for this abnormality.

3 What forms of bladder dysfunction are typically seen in this disorder? Is the neurologic injury static, or does it change (i.e. due to tethering) as the child matures?

4 The voiding cystourethrogram for this child is shown in Fig. 12.10. Urodynamic evaluation reveals an atonic bladder with a capacity of 400 ml. Intravesical pressures remain low up to a volume of 300 ml. What is the most important step that needs to be taken in order to prevent further renal injury?

Discussion

1 This child is seen to have flattened buttocks and a low, short gluteal cleft. Because such children typically have normal sensation and little or no orthopedic deformity in the lower extremities, the underlying lesion is often overlooked. As many as 20% of children with this condition escape detection until the age of 3 or 4 years. The diagnosis of sacral agenesis may be confirmed with a lateral film of the lower spine, which reveals the missing sacral vertebra (Fig. 12.11). MRI of the lumbosacral spine, which is recommended in all patients, consistently reveals a sharp cutoff of the conus at T12.

2 There is an increased association between the development of sacral agenesis and maternal diabetes. Insulin-dependent mothers have up to 1% chance of giving birth to a child with this disorder. Furthermore, 16%

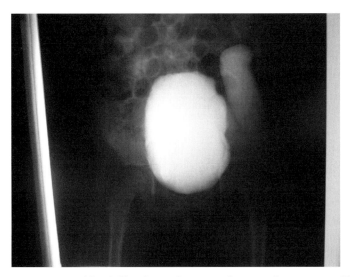

Fig. 12.10 Cystogram of the child with sacral agenesis, showing a large-capacity bladder with high-grade left vesicoureteral reflux.

of children with sacral agenesis have a diabetic mother. However, most cases arise sporadically, and no genetic linkage has been noted. Like all abnormalities of the development of the spine and spinal cord, however, if a parent has one child affected, there is an increased risk of further children being affected with the same condition.

3 Urodynamic testing shows that an almost equal number of individuals manifest a primarily upper (i.e. hypertonic, hyperreflexic) or a primarily lower (i.e. atonic) motor neuron type lesion (35% vs 40%, respectively), while 25% have no sign of bladder dysfunction. The number of affected

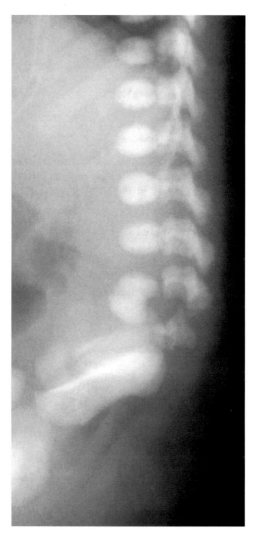

Fig. 12.11 Lateral film of lower spine revealing missing sacral vertebra.

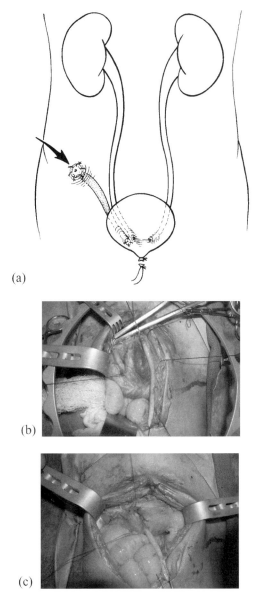

(a)

(b)

(c)

Fig. 12.12 Appendicovesicostomy: extravesical approach. (a) Graphic demonstration of appendix implanted into bladder with abdominal wall stoma for catheterization. (b) Development of muscular flaps on the right lateral aspect of the bladder (appendix shown to the right of bladder incision). (c) Implanted appendix after muscular flaps have been reapproximated to create a submucosal tunnel.

vertebra does not correlate with the type of motor neuron lesion. In contrast to the lesions noted in myelodysplasia or occult spinal cord anomalies, the lesion is stable. It is rare to see signs of progressive denervation, such as a changing urodynamic pattern, in these children as they grow.

4 Treatment with prophylactic antibiotics and surgical correction of the vesicoureteral reflux plays an important role in limiting further injury to the left kidney. However, the most important step that can be taken to limit further renal injury is to improve bladder emptying. Clean intermittent catheterization is an ideal method for achieving this goal. Many children with sacral agenesis are sensate and creation of an alternate route for catheterization, such as an appendicovesicostomy, may improve their compliance with catheterization (Fig. 12.12).

Suggested reading

Boemers T, Van Gool J, deJong T, et al. Urodynamic evaluation of children with caudal regression syndrome (caudal dysplasia sequence). *J Urol.* 1994;151:1038.

Guzman L, Bauer S, Hallet M. The evaluation and management of children with sacral agenesis. *Urology.* 1983;23:506.

Pang D. Sacral agenesis and caudal spinal cord malformations. *Neurosurgery.* 1993;32(5):755–78.

Passarge E, Lenz K. Syndrome of caudal regression in infants of diabetic mothers: observations of further cases. *Pediatrics.* 1966;37:672.

Wilmshurst J, Kelly R, Borzyskowski M. Presentation and outcome of sacral agenesis: 20 years' experience. *Dev Med Child Neurol.* 1999;41:806–12.

13 | Pediatric Urinary Stone Disease

Serdar Tekgül

CASE 1

A 5-year-old boy was admitted with recurrent abdominal pain localized to the left side and radiating to the left lower quadrant with recurrent hematuria and mild lower urinary tract symptoms such as dysuria and urgency. Urinalysis revealed microscopic hematuria with no signs of infection.

1 How would you relate these symptoms in a child to stone disease?
2 What are the common clinical presentations for children with stone disease?
3 What would be the next investigation you would do in such a child?
4 What would be the additional imaging you would do in such a child?
5 How would you manage this child?
6 How useful is extracorporeal shock wave lithotripsy (ESWL) for treating kidney stones in children, and what are the side effects?
7 What is the most probable composition of this stone?
8 How do uric acid stones form, and how should they be managed medically in children?

Discussion

1 Any abdominal pain accompanied with hematuria and urinary symptoms requires additional investigation in the urinary tract to exclude presence of infection and obstruction. One of the common causes of such a clinical setting is urinary calculi.
2 Presentation of urinary calculi in children tends to be age dependent, with symptoms such as flank pain and hematuria being more common in older children. Nonspecific symptoms (e.g. irritability, vomiting) are common in very young children.
   There may be different patterns of clinical presentation.
   • Intense pain that suddenly occurs in the back and radiates downward and centrally toward the lower abdomen or groin. In younger children pain is poorly localized and is often defined as simple abdominal pain.
   • Gross hematuria occurring with or without pain. This is less common in children. Microscopic hematuria may be the sole indicator, and this

is more common in children. Persistent microscopic hematuria, which consists of 5 or more RBCs per high-power field in 3 of 3 consecutive centrifuged urine specimens should be further investigated for urinary stones.

- Infection leading to radiologic imaging that reveals a stone.
- Asymptomatic stones, which are sometimes identified when abdominal imaging is performed for other reasons.

3 Generally, ultrasonography or plain X-ray of the abdomen should be used as the first study. Renal ultrasonography is noninvasive and very effective for identifying stones in the kidney. However, it may fail to show ureteric stones. Many radio-opaque stones can be identified with a simple abdominal plain X-ray examination. If no stone is found but symptoms persist, a noncontrast helical computed tomography (CT) scanning is indicated.

There is nothing remarkable on plain X-ray of the abdomen (Fig. 13.1). Abdominal ultrasound reveals a urinary stone of 6 mm in the left kidney, and there is no dilatation in the collecting system of both kidneys.

4 Since the stone in the kidney is nonopaque and only seen on ultrasound, a noncontrast helical CT scanning will be helpful to confirm the diagnosis of the kidney stone and detect stones in other locations that may have been missed by ultrasound. The most sensitive test for identifying stones in the urinary system is noncontrast helical CT scanning. It is safe and rapid and has been shown to have 97% sensitivity and 96% specificity. Intravenous pyelography is rarely used in children.

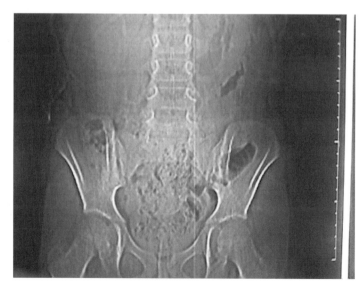

Fig. 13.1

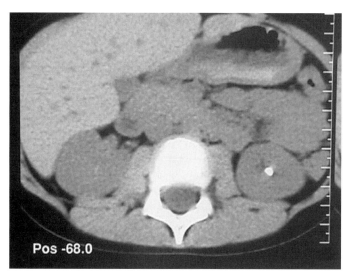

Fig. 13.2

Noncontrast helical CT confirms the presence of a 6-mm stone in the left kidney and reveals an additional 3-mm stone in the distal end of the right ureter (Figs. 13.2 and 13.3).

5 Majority of ureteric stones pass spontaneously. Stone size and location are two most useful parameters in determining the chance of spontaneous passage. A small stone less the 4 mm in size has more than 90% chance

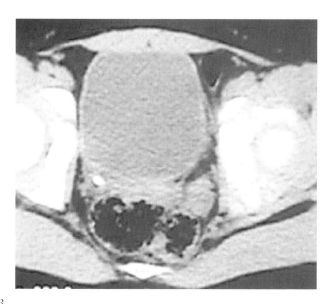

Fig. 13.3

of spontaneous passage. A similar-sized stone located in the upper ureter has a lower chance. Since there is no severe obstruction obviating an intervention, this distal ureteric stone should be managed conservatively.

The kidney stone of 6 mm is too large for spontaneous passage in a child and it should be removed. The best way for removal of stone with a relatively small size like this is extracorporeal shock wave lithotripsy (ESWL). Since it is a nonopaque stone, localization of the stone under ultrasonographic guidance followed by application of ESWL is the best treatment for this child.

6 Nonoperative management of urolithiasis in children carries more risks than in adults. Theoretically, since the tissues are smaller and less mature in children, they are more prone to the local complications of ESWL. Passage of stones following treatment may not be as easy as in adults because of bigger stones relative to the diameter of the urinary tract, and endoscopic manipulation is not always possible in younger patients. Yet, ESWL has been reported successful, with stone-free rates changing from 47% to 96%.

Currently, concerns over the risk of injury to immature kidney and bone tissue have disappeared as several animal studies showed that renal growth and function is not significantly altered after ESWL. Many studies reporting hundreds of children treated by ESWL have confirmed that there is no increased risk of tissue injury altering function and growth. The success rate of ESWL in children has also been found to be similar to adults' success rates. However, the complication rate in children is a little more than in adults and ranges from 1% to 5%. Pulmonary oedema, pulmonary contusion, and urosepsis are possible complications. The lung tissue is susceptible to shock wave energy and it should be protected from direct interaction with shock waves. Metal foams can be used as a barrier to disperse shock wave energy.

ESWL treatment is effective in children with a stone-free rate of 90% and above; some patients may need more than one session of treatment. In different studies, success rates range from 60% to nearly 100% and depend mainly on the stone size, its location, its composition, and type of machines used. The smaller the stone size, the better are the success rates. The ideal stone size for ESWL treatment in adults is less than 2 cm, and this size should be less for children. As the number of stones increases, the stone burden also increases and the clearance rate after ESWL may decrease. An ideal case for ESWL treatment would be a 1–1.5-cm stone located in the renal pelvis.

ESWL can also be used for the treatment of ureteral calculi. The success rates go down for the distal ureteric stones. There may be technical problems with localization and focusing of ureteric stones in children.

7 This is a nonopaque stone, and it is most likely to be a uric acid stone. Plain X-rays are insufficient for uric acid stones, as was the case with this child. Hence renal sonography and spiral CT are used for diagnosis.

Following ESWL treatment the child passed all the fragments of stones within 3–4 days, and the contralateral ureteric stone passed spontaneously within 2 weeks. Analysis of the stones confirmed that they are uric acid stones.

8 Uric acid stones are responsible for urinary calculi in 4–8% of children. Uric acid is the end product of purine metabolism. A uric acid output of more than 10 mg/kg/d is considered to be a sign of hyperuricosuria.

The formation of uric acid stones is dependent mainly on the presence of acidic urinary composition. Uric acid remains in an undissociated and insoluble form at pH of less than 5.8. As the pH becomes more alkaline, uric acid crystals become more soluble and the risk of uric acid stone formation is reduced.

Hyperuricosuria is the main cause of uric acid stone formation in children. In the familial or idiopathic form of hyperuricosuria, children usually have normal serum uric acid levels. In other children, it can be caused by uric acid overproduction secondary to inborn errors of metabolism, myeloproliferative disorders, or other causes of cell breakdown. Although hyperuricosuria is a risk factor for calcium oxalate stone formation in adults, it does not appear to be a significant risk factor in children.

Alkalinization of urine is the mainstay of prevention for uric acid stones. Potassium citrate preparations are useful as alkalinizing agents. Maintaining a urine pH of 6–6.5 is sufficient for prevention of uric acid stones. Dietary purine restriction is often not of major benefit, but increased fluid intake should be encouraged.

If there is severe hyperuricosuria and there is a metabolic condition causing this, allopurinol (10 mg/kg) may be administered to control hyperuricosuria.

CASE 2

A 9-year-old girl was seen after she had episodes of left colicky flank pain with mild hematuria. Plain X-ray of the abdomen shows a left distal ureteric stone of size 0.6 × 1 cm (Fig. 13.4). There is calyceal dilatation in the left collecting system and in the left ureter. She was referred for further management.

1 Would you do further investigations before planning treatment?
2 How would you manage this child?

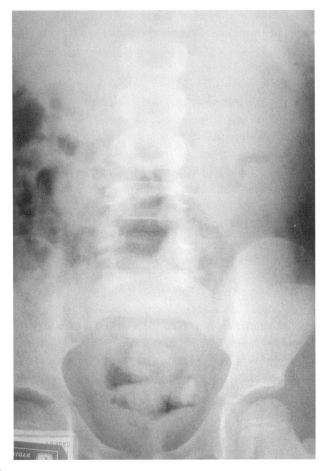

Fig. 13.4

3 How should this patient be evaluated metabolically?

4 What are the causative factors that may play a role in the formation of calcium stones in children, and how should they be managed medically?

Discussion

1 There is usually no need to do more imaging than ultrasound and a plain X-ray of the abdomen if the diagnosis is clear. Intravenous pyelography is rarely used in children. Intravenous urography may be indicated if a congenital anomaly is suspected and there is a need to see the anatomy of the collecting systems and the ureters.

2 Since this stone is too large for spontaneous passage and it is causing obstruction, it should be managed by interventional treatment modalities.

The indications for intervention of a ureteric stone in a child include severe ureteral obstruction, uncontrollable pain, urosepsis, persistent gross hematuria, lack of stone progression, and large stone size.

Distal ureteric stones may be managed by ESWL or intracorporeal lithotripsy using ureterorenoscopy.

ESWL is the least invasive way of treating ureteric stones and may be successful in majority of the cases. Some stones are refractory to ESWL treatment, and there may be technical problems with localization and focusing of ureteric stones in some children.

It has been possible to do ureteroscopy in children using an 11.5F ureteroscope. Different lithotripsy techniques, including ultrasonic, pneumatic, and laser lithotripsy, have all been shown to be safe and effective. There are 8.5F ureteroscopes available, which make use of endoscopic techniques much easier in children. All the studies reporting the use endoscopy for ureteric stones in children have clearly demonstrated that there is no significant risk of ureteric strictures or reflux with this mode of therapy. The success rates in ureteric stones in children with this mode of therapy are higher than with ESWL. Use of extracting forceps or baskets to remove stones from ureters should be avoided as this significantly increases the risk of injury to ureter.

Open surgical removal of a distal ureteric stone in a child is only indicated if other treatments fail, and this is very uncommon.

This patient was managed using an 11F ureteroscope and Holmium-Yag laser lithotripsy. Initially a guidewire was inserted into the ureter, and the ureter was dilated using a balloon dilator inserted over the guidewire. Fragmentation of stone was carried out using Holmium-Yag laser under direct vision. A JJ stent with a string coming out of the urethra was placed. The patient passed majority of fragments within 1–2 days. Two weeks later the JJ stent was removed by pulling the string out; the remaining fragments passed immediately after that and the patient was stone free within 2 weeks after the procedure. (Fig. 13.5) The stone analysis showed that it was a calcium oxalate monohydrate stone.

3 Because of high incidence of predisposing factors for urolithiasis in children and high recurrence rates, a complete metabolic evaluation of every child with urinary stone should be done. Metabolic evaluation includes:
- Family and patient history of metabolic problems.
- Analysis of stone composition.
- Complete blood cell count, electrolytes, blood urea nitrogen, creatinine, calcium, phosphorus, alkaline phosphatase, uric acid, total protein, albumin, PTH (if there is hypercalcemia).

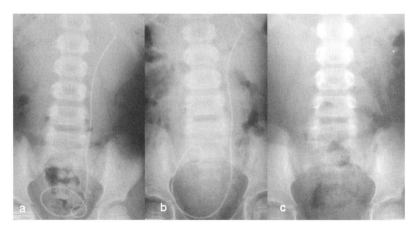

Fig. 13.5

- Spot urinalysis and culture, including ratio of calcium, uric acid, oxalate, cystine, citrate, and magnesium to creatinine.
- Urine tests, including a 24-hour urine collection for calcium, phosphorus, magnesium, oxalate, uric acid citrate, cystine, protein, and creatinine clearance.

In Fig. 13.6, an algorithm is given about how to do metabolic investigation for different stone types and plan medical treatment accordingly.

4 Calcium stones are usually in the form of calcium oxalate stones. Either supersaturation of calcium (hypercalciuria) and oxalate (hyperoxaluria) or decreased concentration of inhibitors such as citrate (hypocitraturia) plays a major role for the calcium oxalate stone formation.

Hypercalciuria

Hypercalciuria is defined by a 24-hour urinary calcium excretion more than 4 mg/kg/d in a child weighing less than 60 kg. In infants younger than 3 months, 5 mg/kg/d is considered the upper limit normal for calcium excretion.

Elevated urinary calcium occurs by three primary mechanisms, as follows:

1 the filtered load of calcium is abnormally increased without an adequate compensatory increase in tubular calcium reabsorption;

2 the filtered calcium load is normal but tubular calcium reabsorption is reduced;

3 the filtered load is increased and the reabsorbed load is reduced.

Hypercalciuria can be classified as idiopathic or secondary. Idiopathic hypercalciuria can be diagnosed when clinical, laboratory, and radiographic

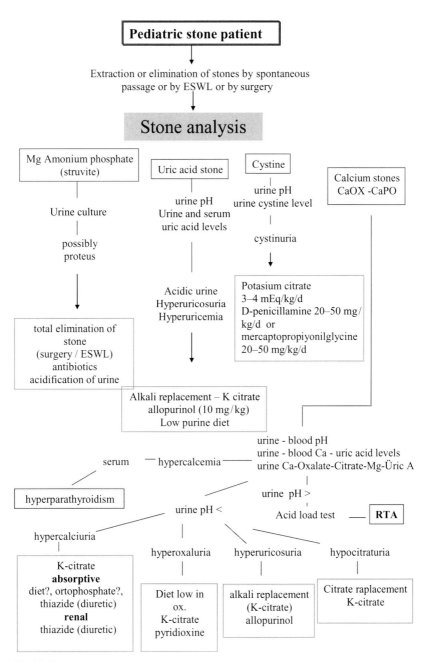

Fig. 13.6

investigations fail to delineate an underlying cause. Secondary hypercalciuria occurs when a known process produces excessive urinary calcium.

As the name implies, the cause of idiopathic hypercalciuria is not known. Several theories have been published, and some data exist to support certain aspects of these theories; however, these theories cannot yet be uniformly applied to a large patient population. Studies looking at metabolic balance have reported increased absorption of calcium from the intestine. In some instances in patients with hypercalciuria, the proportion of calcium excreted into the urine is higher than normal, regardless of dietary intake of calcium. In fact, some patients have been found to have higher than normal urinary calcium despite lower than normal dietary intake, suggesting decreased renal tubular reabsorption.

Idiopathic hypercalcuria is divided into two subtypes.

- *Renal hypercalciuria.* There is decreased reabsorption calcium from the tubule. Therefore there is calcium leak from the kidney (second mechanism mentioned above). It has been postulated that this renal tubular leak is a result of a mutational defect in one or more ion channels.
- *Absorptive hypercalciuria.* There is increased absorption of calcium from the gut. This process has been shown to be independent of vitamin D or a result of increased gut sensitivity to vitamin D. The exact pathogenesis is not known, and this increased uptake may be diet dependent.

Another proposed mechanism for idiopathic hypercalciuria involves an imbalance of calcium deposition and reabsorption in bone that is independent of PTH or vitamin D. It is also quite conceivable that a combination of these factors may be contributing to the high amounts of urinary calcium observed in patients with idiopathic hypercalciuria.

In secondary (hypercalcemic) hypercalciuria, high serum calcium level may be due to increased bone resorption (hyperparathyroidism, hyperthyroidism, immobilization, acidosis, metastatic disease) or gastrointestinal hyper absorption (hypervitaminosis D, sarcoid, milk-alkali syndrome).

A good screening test for hypercalciuria compares the ratio of urinary calcium to creatinine. To validate the screening test, an accurately timed urinalysis should be used to confirm any positive screens. The normal calcium-to-creatinine ratio in children is less than 0.2. If the calculated ratio is higher than 0.2, repeat testing is indicated. One approach is to recheck the ratio at monthly intervals for 2 months. If the follow-up ratios are normal, then no additional testing for hypercalciuria is needed. On the other hand, if the ratio remains elevated, a timed 24-hour urine collection should be obtained and the calcium excretion calculated. The 24-hour calcium excretion test is the criterion standard for the diagnosis of hypercalciuria. If the calcium excretion is higher than 4 mg/kg/d, the diagnosis of hypercalciuria is confirmed and further evaluation is warranted.

Further evaluation includes serum bicarbonate, creatinine, alkaline phosphatase, calcium, magnesium, pH, and parathyroid hormone levels. Freshly voided urine should be measured for bicarbonate and pH. A 24-hour urine collection also should be collected for measurement of calcium, phosphorus, sodium, magnesium, citrate, and oxalate. Meanwhile, dietary manipulations should be tried to normalize urine calcium. Urinary calcium may change with restriction of Na in the diet, especially when it is higher than normal.

The goals of therapy in children with hypercalciuria should be the elimination of symptoms, prevention of renal stone formation, and preservation of kidney function.

Dietary modification is a mandatory part of effective therapy. The main aim of therapy is to increase urinary flow and restriction of dietary sodium. The child should be referred to a dietician to accurately assess daily calcium, animal protein, and sodium intake. A trial of a low-calcium diet can be done transiently to determine if exogenous calcium intake is contributing to the high urinary calcium. However, great caution should be used when trying to restrict calcium intake for long periods.

Hydrochlorothiazide (HCTZ) and other thiazide-type diuretics may be used to treat hypercalciuria. The dose is 1–2 mg/kg/d. Citrate therapy is also useful if citrate levels are low or if hypercalciuria persists despite other therapies.

Hyperoxaluria

Oxalic acid is a metabolite excreted by the kidneys. Only 10–15% of oxalate comes from diet. Normal schoolchildren excrete less than 50 mg/1.73 m^2 a day. This is 4 times more in infants.

Hyperoxaluria may result from increased dietary intake, enteric hyperabsorption (as in short bowel syndrome), or inborn error of metabolism.

In primary hyperoxaluria, one of the two liver enzymes that play a role in the metabolism of oxalate may be deficient. In type I primary hyperoxaluria, alanine:glyoxylate amino transferase enzyme is deficient, and in this case oxalate breakdown is impaired with increase of both oxalate and glycolate. In type II primary hyperoxaluria, D-glycerate dehydrogenase enzyme is deficient, and similarly oxalate breakdown is impaired with increase of both oxalate and L-glycerate. In primary hyperoxaluria there is increased deposition of calcium oxalate in the kidney and in urine. With increased deposition of calcium oxalate in the kidneys, renal failure may ensue resulting in deposition of calcium oxalate in other tissues.

Presentation of primary hyperoxaluria is usually quite early in childhood, and urolithiasis is the common mode of presentation. Symptoms due to deposition of calcium oxalate in other tissues, such as retina, myocardium, and bone marrow, usually become manifest in later stages of the disease.

The diagnosis of severe hyperoxaluria is made on the basis of laboratory findings and clinical symptoms. The definitive diagnosis requires liver biopsy to assay the enzyme activity.

Other forms of hyperoxaluria as mentioned earlier may be due to hyperabsorption of oxalate in inflammatory bowel syndrome, pancreatitis, and short bowel syndrome. It may also be acquired in association with several conditions such as ethylene glycol poisoning, hepatic cirrhosis, renal tubular acidosis, sarcoidosis, cystic fibrosis, and pyridoxine deficiency. Yet, majority of children who have high levels of oxalate excretion in urine may not have any documented metabolic problem or any dietary cause. This is called idiopathic hyperoxaluria, and in this case urine oxalate levels are elevated only mildly.

Treatment of hyperoxaluria consists of promotion of high urine flow and restriction of oxalate in diet. Use of pyridoxine may be useful in reducing urine levels, especially in type I primary hyperoxaluria.

Hypocitraturia

Citrate is a urinary stone inhibitor. Citrate acts by binding to calcium and thus preventing the formation of calcium oxalate or calcium phosphate crystals. Additionally, citrate inhibits the spontaneous nucleation of calcium oxalate. Therefore low urine citrate may be a significant cause for calcium stone disease. Normal citrate values for children are not known. *Hypocitraturia* is excretion of citrate in urine that is less than 320 mg/d for adults. This value may be adjusted for children depending on body size.

Hypocitraturia usually occurs in the absence of any concurrent symptoms or any known metabolic derangements. It can also occur in association with any metabolic acidosis, distal tubular acidosis, or diarrheal syndromes. Environmental factors that lower urinary citrate include a high protein intake and excessive salt intake. Many reports emphasize the significance of hypocitraturia in pediatric calcium stone disease. Presence of hypocitraturia ranges from 30% to 60% in children with calcium stone disease.

Because of the increased stone risk in hypocitraturia, restoration of normal citrate levels is advocated to reduce stone formation. Although there are studies that show citrate replacement therapy reduces stone formation risk in adult population, studies in children are few. Hypocitraturia is treated by potassium citrate at a starting dose of 1 mEq/kg in two divided doses.

Another common cause of hypocitraturia in children is renal tubular acidosis (RTA). Three types of RTA have been described, and only type I RTA is associated with urolithiasis. In type I RTA there is a distal tubular defect in maintaining hydrogen ion gradient. The result is inability to acidify urine to a pH of less than 5.5 despite acid load. The metabolic acidosis caused by this defect will impair renal synthesis of citrate and increase the citrate reabsorpiton, resulting in hypocitraturia. Chronic metabolic acidosis may also lead to hypercalciuria by dissolving calcium salts from the urine and by decreasing renal tubular calcium reabsorption.

Metabolic evaluation of this child revealed that there was only mild hypocitraturia. She was put on citrate replacement therapy (potassium citrate 1 mEq/kg per oral) and advised to increase her daily fluid intake. Her repeat evaluation within 3 months showed that hypocitraturia was corrected and the dose of citrate has been reduced to half of the initial dose (i.e. maintenance dose).

CASE 3

A 9-year-old boy was seen with abdominal pain and repeated proteus infections in the urinary tract. He had been treated with different antibiotics before any imaging study was done. Later his imaging studies showed that he had bilateral staghorn calculi (Fig. 13.7). He has normal renal function tests.

1 What is the most possible stone type in this child?
2 What are infection stones, and how are they formed?
3 How should this child be managed?
4 What is the medical management of infection stones after surgical removal?

Discussion

1 This is most probably an infection stone, as infection stones usually assume a staghorn configuration when located in the kidneys and they are commonly associated with the infection of the urinary tract with urea-splitting organisms like proteus.
2 Infection-related stones constitute nearly 5% of the urinary stones in children. It is reported to be more common in England than many other places. The bacteria that are capable of producing urease enzyme (proteus, klebsiella, and pseudomonas) are responsible for the formation of such stones. Urease converts urea into ammonia and bicarbonate. This alkalinizes the urine and the bicarbonate is further converted into carbonate. In the alkaline environment, triple phosphatase form, and the eventual

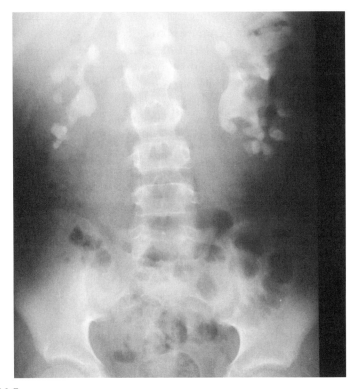

Fig. 13.7

outcome is the supersaturation of magnesium ammonium phosphate and carbonate apatite that lead to stone formation.

Although all infection stones are associated with urea-splitting organism infections, approximately one-half originate from an underlying, readily identifiable anatomic or metabolic defect. Consideration should be given to investigate any congenital problem that causes stasis and infection.

3 In addition to bacterial elimination, stone elimination is essential for treatment because stones may harbor infection inside and antibiotic treatment will not be effective.

Deciding the form of treatment for removal of kidney stones depends on the their number, size, location, and composition and on the anatomy of the urinary tract. Although ESWL is the first choice for many renal stones, an invasive approach would be necessary for larger and complex stones like these. Stone removal can be carried out by means of an open surgical procedure, but percutaneous techniques are being employed more often for the removal of these stones.

For percutaneous renal surgery, identical techniques are used for adults and children. Smaller sized instruments are available (17F nephroscope) for small children. Age does not seem to be a major limitation. Once an access is maintained to the kidney with a proper-sized nephroscope, a variety of instruments can be used to disintegrate (ultrasonic, electrohydraulic, laser lithotripsy) and remove (stone baskets, grasping forceps) the stones. With increasing experience, not only success rates have increased but also the complications have become very insignificant. Stone-free rates around 90% have been reported in many series with this technique. There were no significant complications, but some patients needed a secondary look through a preexisting nephrostomy tube.

Although most of the stones in children can be managed by ESWL and endoscopic techniques, open surgery would be necessary in some situations. Very young children with large stones and/or congenitally obstructed systems that also need surgical correction are good candidates for open stone surgery. Severe orthopedic deformities may limit positioning for endoscopic procedures, and open surgery would also be a necessity for such children. Sometimes, when the staghorn stone is too large and complicated with many branches, open surgical approach with a radial anatrophic nephrolithotomy may be preferred to a percutaneous approach, which would need more than 2–3 accesses to the kidney.

Complete removal of infection stones is necessary, since residual fragments may harbor infection, which may regenerate stone formation.

This child has undergone a combination of different techniques for the removal of stones. First, a percutaneous nephrolithotomy was performed on the right side, and a remaining 10-mm stone was managed by ESWL. Later, the left-kidney stones were removed by open surgery with the anatrophic nephrolithotomy technique. The child was stone-free 6 weeks after the initiation of the therapy. The stones were struvite stones (Figs. 13.8).

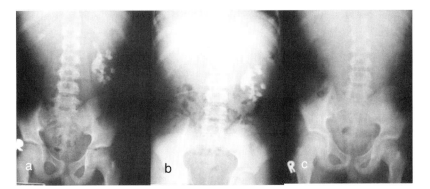

Fig. 13.8

4 All children with known infection stones should undergo a complete metabolic evaluation to exclude the presence of underlying metabolic disorders. In patients having no metabolic disorders other than urinary tract infection, medical management of infection is essential.

Patients should be monitored closely for recurrence of infection; when identified, the infection should be promptly treated.

Suggested reading

Barratt TM, Duffey PG. *Nephrocalcinosis and Urolithiasis*. 4th ed. Philadelphia: Lippincott-Raven; 1999.

Diamond DA, Rickwood AM, Lee PH, Johnston JH. Infection stones in children: a twenty-seven-year review. *Urology*. 1994;43:525–7.

Drach GW. Metabolic evaluation of paediatric patients with stones. *Urol Clin North Am.* 1995;22:95–100.

Harmon EP, Neal DE, Thomas R. Paediatric urolithiasis: review of research and current management. *Pediatr Nephrol*. Aug 1994;8(4):508–12.

Kaji DM, Xie HW, Hardy BE, et al. The effects of extracorporeal shock wave lithotripsy on renal growth, function and arterial blood pressure in an animal model. *J Urol*. 1991;146(2 pt 2):544–7.

Langman CB, Moore ES. Paediatric urolithiasis. In: Edelmann CM Jr, ed. *Paediatric Kidney Disease*. Vol 2. Philadelphia: Lippincott; 1992:2005–14.

Schenkman NA, Stoller ML. Urinary stone disease. In: Rakel RE, ed. *Conn's Current Therapy*. 51st ed. Philadelphia: Saunders; 1999:741.

Stapleton FB. What is the appropriate evaluation and therapy for children with hypercalciuria and hematuria? *Semin Nephrol*. 1998;18:359–60.

Thomas R, Frentz JM, Harmon E, et al. Effect of extracorporeal shock wave lithotripsy on renal function and body height in paediatric patients. *J Urol*. 1992;148(3 pt 2):1064–66.

Thomas R, Ortenberg J, Lee BR, et al. Safety and efficacy of paediatric ureteroscopy for management of calculous disease. *J Urol*. 1993;149(5):1082–4.

14 | Genitourinary Tumors

Laurence Baskin and Hubert S. Swana

CASE 1

A nine-year-old boy presents with a painless testicular mass (Fig. 14.1).

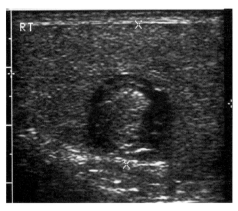

Fig. 14.1 Testicular ultrasound from a 9-year-old boy with a testicular mass.

1 Discuss the epidemiology of testicular tumors in children.
2 Discuss the most common pediatric testicular tumors.
3 Discuss clinical presentation, diagnosis, and workup of testicular masses.
4 Discuss pathology and staging.
5 Briefly discuss the treatment for prepubertal testicular tumors.

Discussion

1 Testicular tumors in infants and children are relatively uncommon. They account for 1–2% of all pediatric solid tumors. The incidence is between 0.5 and 2.0 cases per 100,000 boys. This is less than 5.4 cases per 100,000 adults. Germ cell tumors account for only 60–75% of testicular tumors in children, whereas 95% of adult testicular tumors are germ cell tumors.
2 Yolk sac tumor is the most common pediatric germ cell tumor. Some reports suggest that the incidence of mature teratoma may exceed that of yolk sac tumor. Seminoma and teratocarcinoma occur less often. Gonadal stromal tumors, such as Leydig cell tumor, Sertoli cell tumor, and juvenile

165

granulosa cell tumor, are also seen. Gonadoblastoma is seen with intersex disorders, usually in phenotypic females with intra-abdominal streak gonads or testes.

3 Most commonly, children present with an enlarging painless mass. Leydig cell tumors can be a cause of precocious puberty and gynecomastia. Ultrasonography is helpful in assessing scrotal pathology. Solid intratesticular tumors can be distinguished from paratesticular masses. Tumor markers should be assessed both pre- and postoperatively. Tumors that contain yolk sac elements produce alpha-fetoprotein (AFP). Beta human chorionic gonadotropin (HCG) is not commonly elevated in prepubertal patients. Both mixed germ cell tumors and embryonal tumors can produce beta HCG. Computed tomography (CT) of the retroperitoneum and chest is helpful for staging.

4 The Children's Cancer Group (CCG)/Pediatric Oncology Group (POG) intergroup study uses the following system:

Stage I Tumor limited to testis is completely resected. Complete resection is possible by high inguinal orchiectomy. An appropriate decline in tumor markers is seen and is negative.

Stage II Microscopic residual disease is seen in the scrotum or spermatic cord. Tumor markers remain elevated after an appropriate half-life interval. Tumor rupture or scrotal biopsy is performed prior to complete orchiectomy.

Stage III Retroperitoneal lymph node involvement (>2 cm) is present. There is no visible evidence of visceral or extra-abdominal involvement.

Stage IV Distant metastases are present including liver.

5 Treatment for yolk sac tumors begins with radical orchiectomy. Stage I patients are closely followed with serial AFP measurement and periodic imaging of the retroperitoneum and chest. Routine retroperitoneal lymph node dissection is not performed. Patients of stage II and higher are treated with chemotherapy. Patients with persistent elevated AFP or persistent retroperitoneal mass may require retroperitoneal lymph node dissection.

Testicle sparing surgery after frozen section confirmation can be employed to cure children with teratoma, epidermoid cysts, and Leydig cell tumors. The treatment of gonadoblastoma involves removal of the gonad. Streak gonads should be removed because of risk of malignant degeneration.

Suggested reading

Grady RW. Current management of prepubertal yolk sac tumors of the testis. *Urol Clin North Am.* 2000;27(3):503–508.

Levin HS. Tumors of the testis in intersex syndromes. *Urol Clin North Am.* 2000;27(3): 543–51.

Ritchey ML. Pediatric oncology. In: Campbell MF, Walsh PC, eds. *Campbell's Urology.* 6th ed. Philadelphia: Saunders; 1996.

Synder HM III, Cooper CS. Pediatric neoplasia. In: Weiss RM, George NJR, O'Reilly PH, eds. *Comprehensive Urology.* London, UK: Harcourt Press; 2000.

CASE 2

A 3-year-old girl presents with a new abdominal mass (Fig. 14.2).

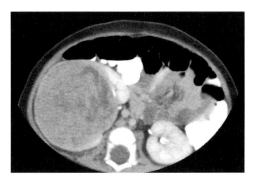

Fig. 14.2 CT scan of a 3-year-old girl with a painless abdominal mass.

1 Discuss the epidemiology of Wilms tumor.
2 Discuss the genetics of Wilms tumor.
3 Discuss the clinical presentation of Wilms tumor.
4 Discuss the pathology and staging of Wilms tumor.
5 Discuss the differences between National Wilms Tumor Study Group (NWTSG) and International Society of Pediatric Oncology (SIOP) protocols for treating children with Wilms tumor.
6 Describe non-Wilms tumors of the kidney.

Discussion

1 Wilms tumor or nephroblastoma is the most common childhood abdominal malignancy. Wilms tumor affects approximately 10 children per million before the age of 15 years. Approximately 450–500 new cases are diagnosed each year in the United States. In 5–10% of cases, both kidneys are affected. The median age at diagnosis is approximately 3.5 years. Wilms tumor appears to be more common in African and African American children than Caucasian or Asian children. The male-to-female ratio is 0.92:1.00. For patients with bilateral disease, the male-to-female ratio is 0.60:1.00.

2 The first Wilms tumor suppressor gene *WT1* was cloned in 1990. *WT1* encodes a transcription factor critical to normal kidney and gonadal development. The *WT1* gene has now been shown to be the specific target of mutations and deletion events in a subset of sporadic Wilms tumors, as well as in the germline of some children (e.g. those with Denys–Drash syndrome) with genetic predisposition to this cancer. A second Wilms tumor predisposing gene has been identified (but is not yet cloned) telomeric of *WT1*, at 11p15.

3 Wilms tumor most commonly presents with a painless abdominal mass. Some patients present with hematuria, hypertension, or fever. Patients who experience acute hemorrhage can present with hypotension, anemia, and fever. Patients with pulmonary metastases can present with respiratory symptoms. Several associated congenital anomalies have been reported including aniridia, hypospadias, cryptorchidism, and hemihypertrophy. Aniridia and Wilms tumor are seen together in the WAGR syndrome (Wilms tumor, aniridia, genital anomalies, and mental retardation). Denys–Drash syndrome is the specific association of Wilms tumor with male pseudohermaphrotidism and renal mesangial sclerosis. Beckwith–Weidemann syndrome consists of organomegaly (macroglossia, hepatomegaly) or hemihypertrophy and Wilms tumor.

4 A typical Wilms tumor has three histologic components: stromal, epithelial, and blastemal (Fig. 14.3). Anaplasia is seen in a small number of patients and portends a worse prognosis.

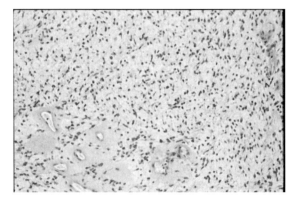

Fig. 14.3 Histology of Wilms tumor demonstrating a predominantly stromal tumor with blastemal elements in the upper right field and epithelial elements in the lower left corner.

Staging of Wilms Tumor

Stage I The tumor is limited to the kidney and completely excised. The renal capsule is intact and the tumor is not ruptured prior to removal. There is no residual tumor.

Stage II The tumor extends through renal capsule but is still completely excised. Local spillage confined to flank may have occurred. Biopsy may have occurred. Extra renal vessels may contain tumor thrombus or be infiltrated by tumor.

Stage III There is a nonhematogenous residual tumor, gross or microscopic, confined to the abdomen and lymph node involvement within abdomen or pelvis, peritoneal implants, diffuse peritoneal spillage not confined to flank, and residual tumor.

Stage IV Hematogenous metastases (e.g. liver, lung bone, brain) or lymph node metastases outside the abdominopelvic region are observed.

Stage V At diagnosis, bilateral renal involvement is found. Each side should be staged individually according to the above criteria.

5 Both NWTSG and SIOP protocols have improved survival for patients with Wilms tumor. In Europe (SIOP) biopsy and preoperative chemotherapy is administered prior to attempts at surgical extirpation. Advantages include tumor shrinkage and easier surgical removal with decreased tumor rupture. Disadvantages include less precision in staging. In North America (NWTSG) a surgical approach is generally used, followed by chemotherapy with or without radiation therapy. In patients with bilateral tumors under NWTSG protocols, preoperative chemotherapy is employed.

6 Congenital mesoblastic nephroma. These generally occur in patients under 3 months of age and are cured by nephrectomy alone. Clear cell sarcoma of the kidney has a tendency to metastasize to bone and brain. They require combination radiation and doxorubicin-based chemotherapy. Lower stage tumors have a good prognosis. Rhabdoid tumor of the kidney is a very aggressive and lethal tumor. It is chemoresistant, and most patients with advanced disease do not survive. Renal cell carcinoma in children is more common in the second decade of life. As with adults, complete surgical resection is crucial for cure.

Suggested reading

Breslow N, Olshan A, Beckwith JB. Epidemiology of Wilms tumor. *Med Pediatr Oncol.* 1993;21(3):172–81.

Coppes MJ, Pritchard-Jones K. Principles of Wilms' tumor biology. *Urol Clin North Am.* 2000;27(3):423–33.

Egeler RM, Wolff JE, Anderson RA. Long-term complications and post-treatment follow-up of patients with Wilms' tumor. *Semin Urol Oncol.* 1999;17(1):55–61.

CASE 3

A two-year-old boy presents with gross hematuria and progressive obstructive symptoms (Fig. 14.4).

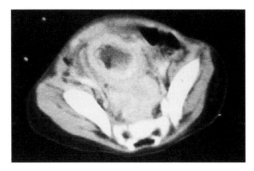

Fig. 14.4 CT scan of the patient with prostatic rhabdomyosarcoma. He presented with hematuria.

1 Discuss epidemiology of rhabdomyosarcoma (RMS).
2 Discuss the clinical presentation of RMS.
3 Discuss the histology of RMS.
4 Detail the staging of RMS.
5 Describe treatment for RMS.
6 Discuss the survival rates of RMS.

Discussion

1 Rhabdomyosarcoma (RMS) is the most common sarcoma of childhood. Rhabdomyosarcoma comprises about 15% of all childhood solid tumors. One fifth of these arise from the urinary tract. The incidence of genitourinary RMS is 0.5–0.7 cases per million in children under 15 years of age. RMS is more common in males than females (1.4:1) and in Caucasians than African Americans (2.3:1). The most common genitourinary sites are prostate, bladder, and paratestis.

2 Presenting symptoms depend on the organ of origin. Patients with prostatic or bladder involvement may present with irritative symptoms followed by hematuria. Enlarging prostatic primaries may cause urinary retention or constipation. Girls with vaginal primaries may present with vaginal discharge, bleeding, or visible tumor mass at the introitus. Patients with paratesticular masses usually present with a painless, enlarging scrotal mass.

3 Embryonal rhabdomyosarcoma accounts for 60% of all rhabdomyosarcomas. The cells resemble fetal skeletal muscle and possess abundant eosinophilic cytoplasm. One variant of embryonal RMS is botryoides type. Grossly they are polypoid and arise from hollow organs or cavities such as vagina or bladder. Spindle cell sarcomas are an embryonal variant with an excellent prognosis, usually seen in males with low stage paratesticular primaries. Alveolar RMS is the second most common histologic subtype (20%). Its multiple small round cells with scant eosinophilic cytoplasm are arranged in architecture similar to pulmonary alveoli. It has a higher rate of recurrence; 10 to 20% of cases are undifferentiated (anaplastic) and are associated with a worse prognosis.

4 Over the past several decades the staging of RMS has evolved. Prior staging systems relied on extent of surgical resection for classification. The collaborative efforts of the Intergroup Rhabdomyosarcoma Study Group have led to the development of a staging system (IRS-IV) that includes pretreatment stage (tumor, node, and metastases) while considering site of origin. Favorable GU sites include the vulva and vagina. Unfavorable sites include the prostate, bladder, and uterus.

5 The management of bladder and prostate tumors has evolved. Most children are initially treated with chemotherapy with or without radiation therapy. Surgery is reserved for residual disease. With current regimens, 60% of patients can preserve their bladder. Radical cystectomy and radical prostatectomy are reserved for select cases.

Initial intervention for paratesticular RMS includes radical orchiectomy. Children older than 10 years should undergo ipsilateral retroperitoneal lymph node dissection. They then receive chemotherapy with or without radiotherapy. Children with RMS of the vagina and uterus receive chemotherapy before any attempt at resection.

6 Survival rates have improved. The overall survival rate for patients with RMS is 75% (long-term survival). Paratesticular and vaginal RMS have the best prognosis (90%). Only 40% of patients with uterine tumors survive.

Suggested reading

Barr FG. Molecular genetics and pathogenesis of rhabdomyosarcoma. *J Pediatr Hematol Oncol.* 1997;19(6):483–91.

Flamant F, Rodary C, Rey A, et al. Treatment of non-metastatic rhabdomyosarcomas in childhood and adolescence. Results of the second study of the International Society of Paediatric Oncology: MMT84. *Eur J Cancer.* 1998;34(7):1050–62.

Pappo AS, Shapiro DN, Crist WM. Rhabdomyosarcoma. Biology and treatment. *Pediatr Clin North Am.* 1997;44(4):953–72.

CASE 4

An 8-month-old boy is brought in to the pediatrician's office. His parents have noticed a new abdominal mass (Fig. 14.5).

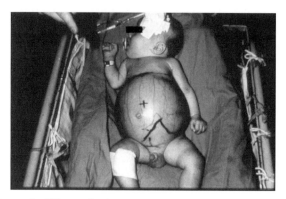

Fig. 14.5 A 8-month-old boy with a large abdominal mass.

1 What is your differential and most likely diagnosis?
2 Discuss common presenting signs and symptoms.
3 Describe the initial workup.
4 Discuss molecular and biochemical prognostic factors.
5 Discuss the staging.
6 Describe risk-based treatment.

Discussion

1 Pediatric abdominal masses can either be malignant or benign. Malignant tumors include neuroblastoma, Wilms tumor, rhabdomyosarcoma, hepatoblastoma, lymphoma, lymphosarcoma, and renal cell sarcoma. Benign abdominal masses can be due to multicystic dysplastic kidney, hydronephrosis, polycystic kidney, congenital mesoblastic nephroma, mesenteric cysts, intestinal duplication cyst, or splenomegaly.

Neuroblastoma is the most common solid tumor of infancy. It is a malignancy of the sympathetic nervous system that arises from neuroblasts (pluripotent sympathetic cells). During development these cells invaginate, migrate along the neuraxis, and populate the sympathetic ganglia, adrenal medulla, and other sites. The sites of disease correlate with this distribution pattern. Prognosis and treatment recommendations are based on age, stage, and molecular characteristics. Infants younger than 1 year have a good prognosis, even in the presence of metastatic disease. Unfortunately, a majority (70–80%) of patients older than 1 year present with metastatic disease, usually to lymph nodes, liver, bone, and brain. Even with aggressive multimodal therapy the cure rates for these children is only 50%.

2 Signs and symptoms depend on the sites of involvement and extent of disease Symptoms can include abdominal masses, with or without pain, emesis, irritability, weight loss, anorexia, and fatigue. Hypertension due to renal artery compression is uncommon. Patients with advanced-stage disease and bone involvement present with bone pain, limping, and pathologic fractures. Periorbital ecchymosis and proptosis are secondary to metastatic disease to the orbits. Spinal cord compression from tumors arising from parasympathetic ganglia can result in weakness, bladder dysfunction, bowel dysfunction, and even paralysis. Skin lesions in the form of subcutaneous blue nodules can also be seen.

3 Staging and treatment planning requires thorough evaluation.

Laboratory studies should include complete blood count, ferritin levels, serum lactate dehydrogenase, electrolytes, creatinine, calcium, magnesium, liver function tests, and timed urine collections for catecholamines (vanillylmandelic acid and homovanillic acid).

Imaging studies should include chest and abdominal radiographs. Skeletal surveys may be helpful in documenting disease extent. Bone scanning with technetium (Tc-99) can help in evaluation of metastatic bone disease. Computed tomography will help assess primary tumor location and disease extent. Magnetic resonance imaging is very useful in assessment of cord compression and intraspinal disease and vascular involvement. $I^{121/131}$-methyliodobenzylguanidine (MIBG) scanning also can be helpful in primary disease assessment and follow-up.

4 Elevated neuron-specific enolase (>200 ng/ml), serum ferritin (143 ng/ml) and lactic dehydrogenase (1500 ng/dl) all signify a poorer prognosis. Histologic criteria developed by Shimada can differentiate patients with favorable histology and unfavorable histology by looking at the presence or absence of stroma, mitotic karyorrhexis, and degree of differentiation. Amplification of the *n*-myc oncogene is associated with rapid tumor progression and poor prognosis. Flow cytometry can also provide useful prognostic information. Diploid or tetraploid tumors are highly aggressive. Near-triploidy is associated with a favorable prognosis.

5 Older classification systems have been replaced by an international staging system. This staging system, which incorporates the patient's age, when combined with molecular data allows for risk stratification and forms the basis for treatment.

6 Low-risk patients have a greater than 90% three-year survival with surgical excision alone. Intermediate risk patients receive a combination of surgery and chemotherapy. Selected patients also receive radiation therapy. High-risk patients require even more intense treatment, which includes chemotherapy, radiation, and surgery for diagnosis, tumor debulking, or, when possible, complete resection. Some may also derive benefit from myeloablative therapy and bone marrow transplantation, but morbidity is significant. Three-year survival rates average between 10-40%.

Suggested reading

Brodeur GM, Castleberry RP. Neuroblastoma. In: Pizzo PA, Poplack DG, eds. *Principles and Practices of Pediatric Oncology*. 3rd ed. Philadelphia: Lippincott-Raven; 1997:769.

Perez CA, Matthay KK, Atkinson JB, et al. Biologic variables in the outcome of stages I and II neuroblastoma treated with surgery as primary therapy: a children's cancer group study. *J Clin Oncol*. 2000;18(1):18–26.

Shimada H, Ambros IM, Dehner LP, et al. Terminology and morphologic criteria of neuroblastic tumors: recommendations by the International Neuroblastoma Pathology Committee. *Cancer*. 1999;86(2):349–63.

15 | Female Genital Anomalies

Duncan T. Wilcox

CASE 1

A 3-year-old girl has been brought by the parents with a history that, while changing the nappies, her mother noticed abnormal female genitalia.

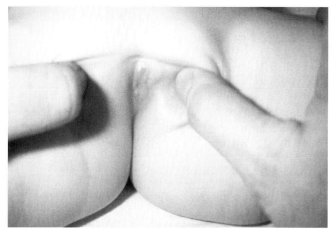

Fig. 15.1

1 Describe the findings in the above picture.
2 What is the possible diagnosis and differential diagnosis?
3 What are the other modes of presentation?
4 What are the different treatment options available?

Discussion

1 The picture shows fused labia. The urethral meatus and vaginal introitus are completely hidden under the labia.
2 This condition is called fused labia or labial adhesions and is common in newborns and during early childhood. Trauma, superficial infection, and chemical irritation from the perineal wetness have been implicated. Denudation of the delicate, poorly estrogenized labial epithelium allows

subsequent agglutination. A careful, gentle, and detailed examination is important to reveal the anatomy. Sometimes the complete labial fusion without the thin membrane results in a single orifice and should raise the suspicion of a urogenital sinus. Vulval changes with labial adhesions raise the possibility of sexual abuse.

3 Usually the adhesions are asymptomatic. The urine trapped in these labial folds may act as a source for urinary tract infection (UTI), postmicturition dribbling, or urinary incontinence.

4 In general, labial adhesions do not warrant treatment and resolve on their own during puberty under the influence of the estrogen. Symptomatic or bothersome adhesions can be treated with regular application of estrogen cream (0.1%) 3 times daily for at least 2 weeks. After separation, Vaseline should be applied daily for another month. Rarely, the adhesions need separation under anesthesia. There is a high chance of recurrence.

Suggested reading

Bacon JL. Prepubertal labial adhesions: evaluation of a referral population. *Am J Obstet Gynecol.* 2002;187(2):327–31; discussion 332.

McCann J, Voris J, Simon M. Labial adhesions and posterior fourchette injuries in childhood sexual abuse. *Am J Dis Child.* 1988;142:659–63.

Nurzia MJ, Eickhorst KM, Ankem MK, Barone JG. The surgical treatment of labial adhesions in pre-pubertal girls. *J Pediatr Adolesc Gynecol.* 2003;16(1):21–3.

Opipari AW Jr. Management quandary. Labial agglutination in a teenager. *J Pediatr Adolesc Gynecol.* 2003;16(1):61–2.

Papagianni M, Stanhope R. Labial adhesions in a girl with isolated premature thelarche: the importance of estrogenization. *J Pediatr Adolesc Gynecol.* 2003;16(1):31–2.

Thibaud E, Duflos C. Plea for child: labial agglutination should not be treated [in French]. *Arch Pediatr.* 2003;10(5):465–6.

CASE 2

A 14-year-old girl is complaining of recurrent cyclical abdominal pain. A detailed history reveals she is still not menstruating. Examination findings are shown in Fig. 15.2.

1 What is the probable diagnosis? And what is the other mode of presentation?

2 What is the embryological reason for this anomaly?

3 What imaging is required for diagnosis?

4 What is the treatment option?

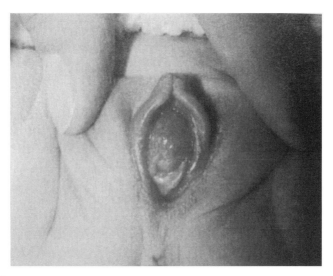

Fig. 15.2

Discussion

1 This condition is called as imperforate hymen. The cyclical pain is due to the accumulation of the menstruating fluid into the vagina. This condition can present as a hydrocolpos or mucocolpos (abdominal mass) due to the accumulation of secretions (blood, mucus) in the vagina. In the newborn period this may present as a hydrocolpos due to accumulation of secretions under the influence of the maternal estrogen.

2 It results from the failure of distal canalization of the vaginal plate at the junction between the urogenital sinus and the vagina.

3 The diagnosis is clinical, but an ultrasound scan of the abdomen is helpful to see the hydrometrocolpos, seen as a pelvic cyst. Sometimes there is mild bilateral hydronephrosis due to secondary compression.

4 Incision of the hymeneal membrane (hymnectomy) is adequate to drain the secretion and treat this condition. There are recent reports of treatment of this condition with balloon dilation.

Suggested reading

Ali A, Cetin C, Nedim C, Kazim G, Cemalettin A. Treatment of imperforate hymen by application of Foley catheter. *Eur J Obstet Gynecol Reprod Biol.* 2003;106(1):72–5

Joki-Erkkila MM, Heinonen PK. Presenting and long-term clinical implications and fecundity in females with obstructing vaginal malformations. *J Pediatr Adolesc Gynecol.* 2003;16(5):307–12.

Liang CC, Chang SD, Soong YK. Long-term follow-up of women who underwent surgical correction for imperforate hymen. *Arch Gynecol Obstet*. 2003;269(1):5–8.

Lim YH, Ng SP, Jamil MA. Imperforate hymen: report of an unusual familial occurrence. J Obstet Gynaecol Res. 2003;29(6):399–401.

Wall EM, Stone B, Klein BL. Imperforate hymen: a not-so-hidden diagnosis. *Am J Emerg Med*. 2003;21(3):249–50.

CASE 3

A 2-year-old girl is referred by the general practitioner, because the parents have noticed a prolapsing interlabial mass. Examination reveals a soft red-coloured cystic mass prolapsing through the introitus.

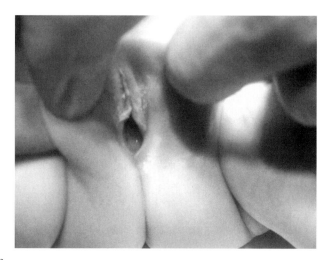

Fig. 15.3

1 What is the likely diagnosis, and what is the differential diagnosis?

2 What further imaging is needed?

3 How do you treat this girl, and what are the different options available for the other interlabial masses?

Discussion

1 The differential diagnosis of the interlabial mass are prolapsed ureterocele, prolapsed urethra, urethral polyp, paraurethral cyst, and sarcoma botryoides.

    Large ectopic ureteroceles associated with the upper pole of the duplex kidney are prone to prolapse. The prolapsed ureterocele is usually cystic and covered with pink bladder mucosa.

Prolapsed urethra usually presents with blood spotting in addition to the mass and associated lower tract urinary symptoms. The urethral mucosa is congested and friable and appears as a purple doughnut encircling the urethral meatus.

Urethral polyps of the posterior urethra are a rare type of interlabial mass and are also associated with blood spotting.

Congenital paraurethral cysts are rare and result from the ductal obstruction of the skene's paraurethral gland. These are smooth, soft, and whitish and sometimes displace the urethral meatus.

Sarcoma botryoides is a polypoid form of embryonal rhabdomyosarcoma. The tumour arises in the bladder, vagina, or, rarely, the uterus. The polypoid tissue resembles a "bunch of grapes".

2 An ultrasound scan of the urinary tract and pelvis is important. Depending on the definitive diagnosis, further imaging is needed for the management.

Ectopic ureteroceles are usually associated with duplex kidneys; a micturating cystourethrogram to asses the vesicoureteral reflux and a DMSA scan to evaluate the differential function of duplex kidney are necessary.

Prolapsing urethral mucosa, urethral polyp, and paraurethral cyst do not need further investigations.

Sarcoma botryoides needs a cystovaginoscopy and biopsy to prove the diagnosis. A computed tomography (CT) scan of the abdomen, pelvis, and chest is needed for the staging of the disease.

3 Prolapsed ureterocele require a cystoscopy and puncturing of the ureterocele as an immediate treatment and then a definitive treatment depending on the function of the upper moiety. The upper moiety of the duplex kidney with this ureterocele is usually nonfunctioning and necessitates an upper pole heminephrectomy (open or laparoscopic). The risk of urinary incontinence should be explained in this group of patients because of associated poor development of the bladder neck.

The symptoms of the prolapsed urethra usually resolve with topical estrogen cream, but persistence of this may need surgical excision of the prolapsed mucosa.

The urethral polyp needs a simple excision and fulguration of the base.

A paraurethral cyst found in a newborn spontaneously drains within a few months. If it persists, it needs a simple aspiration or incision and marsupialization.

Sarcoma botryoides or embryonal rhabdomyosarcoma responds to chemotherapy well. Reassessment of the tumour burden after chemotherapy and limited resection (organ preserving) surgery are recommended. The single polypoid lesion of the cervix has a good prognosis, and simple excision is enough to treat this condition.

Suggested reading

Behtash N, Mousavi A, Tehranian A, Khanafshar N, Hanjani P. Embryonal rhabdomyosarcoma of the uterine cervix: case report and review of the literature. *Gynecol Oncol.* 2003;91(2):452–5.

Hicks BA, Hensle TW, Burbige KA, et al. Bladder management in children with genitourinary sarcoma. *J Pediatr Surg.* 1993;28(8):1019–22.

Klee LW, Rink RC, Gleason PE, Ganesan GS, Mitchell ME, Heifetz SA. Urethral polyp presenting as interlabial mass in young girls. *Urology.* 1993;41(2):132–3.

Miller MA, Cornaby AJ, Nathan MS, Pope A, Morgan RJ. Prolapsed ureterocele: a rare vulval mass. *Br J Urol.* 1994;73(1):109–10.

Nussbaum AR, Lebowitz RL. Interlabial masses in little girls: review and imaging recommendations. *AJR Am J Roentgenol.* 1983;141(1):65–71.

Sharifi-Aghdas F, Ghaderian N. Female paraurethral cysts: experience of 25 cases. *BJU Int.* 2004;93(3):353–6.

CASE 4

A newborn girl with a lower abdominal cystic swelling and abnormal perineal anatomy is referred by the pediatrician. On clinical examination there was a lower abdominal swelling. Examination of perineum revealed a single opening.

1 Describe the findings (clinical and radiological) see Fig. 15.4?
2 What are the likely diagnosis and differential diagnosis?
3 What other systems should you examine to complete the evaluation, and why?
4 What is the emergency treatment for this condition?
5 Describe the definitive management of this condition.
6 What information will you give the parents regarding the long-term consequences?

Discussion

1 The clinical picture shows a single perineal opening, and there is no separate opening of the urethra, vagina, and the anus. The genitogram shows a common channel.
2 The likely diagnosis in this case is cloaca, i.e. a single channel of the genital tract, the urinary tract, and the rectum. The abdominal swelling (hydrometrocolpos) is the distended vagina due to the retrograde filling by the urine and secretions from the endometrium under influence of the maternal estrogen. In patients with urogenital (UG) sinus there is a common channel of the urethra and the vagina but a separate opening for the

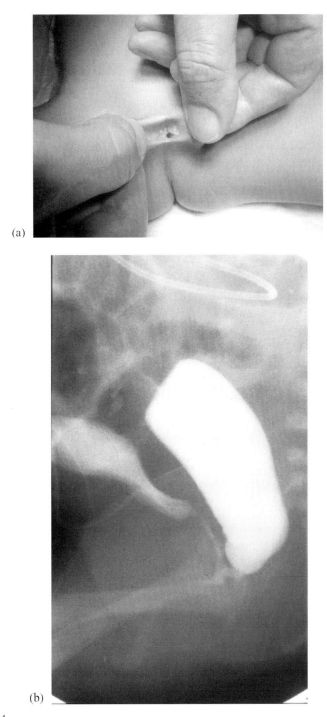

(a)

(b)

Fig. 15.4

anus. UG sinus abnormalities may occur with congenital adrenal hyperplasia (CAH). With widespread expertise in antenatal scan, cloaca can be diagnosed antenatally.

3 A complete physical examination to rule out dysmorphic features of the syndromes is important. Cloaca is associated with a multiorgan system involvement: cardiac (10%), respiratory (5%), spinal (30%), renal (30%), and limb anomalies. Echocardiography, spinal and renal ultrasound, and urodynamic studies of the bladder are mandatory to rule out these abnormalities.

4 Once the child is stable, she needs a defunctioning colostomy and cystovaginoscopy with suprapubic drainage of hydrometrocolpos for decompression. This condition is best managed at a tertiary center with multidisciplinary team approach. Once the fluid is drained from the hydrometrocolpos and natural voiding commences, both catheters can be removed. Rarely, if voiding is not possible, then a clean intermittent catheterization should be started to drain the common channel.

5 The definitive management is deferred until 1 year of age. The stepwise approach involves the initial stage of the posterior sagittal approach to mobilize the UG sinus with the pull-through (posterior sagittal anorecto-vaginourethroplasty, or PSARVUP) to create the neourethral, vaginal, and anal opening. After an interval of about 3–6 months the defunctioning colostomy is closed.

6 This complex abnormality is rare, occurring in 1 in 40,000–50,000 live births. The surgical repair is extremely complex, but the results are satisfactory. Eighty percent of the patients are socially continent of urine and 60% are fecally continent. Urinary incontinence is due to the underlying spinal or bladder abnormality. Fifty percent of these patients develop chronic renal failure due to the underlying renal abnormalities. The recent literature reports a satisfactory long-term outcome regarding sexual function.

Suggested reading

De Gennaro M, Rivosecchi M, Lucchetti MC, Silveri M, Fariello G, Schingo P. The incidence of occult spinal dysraphism and the onset of neurovesical dysfunction in children with anorectal anomalies. *Eur J Pediatr Surg.* 1994;4(suppl 1):12–14.

Krstic ZD, Lukac M, Lukac R, Smoljanic Z, Vukadinovic V, Varinac D. Surgical treatment of cloacal anomalies *Pediatr Surg Int.* 2001;17(4):329–33.

Hendren WH. Cloaca, the most severe degree of imperforate anus: experience with 195 cases. *Ann Surg.* 1998;228(3):331–46

Nakayama DK, Snyder HM, Schnaufer L, Ziegler MM, Templeton JM Jr, Duckett JW Jr. Posterior sagittal exposure for reconstructive surgery for cloacal anomalies. *J Pediatr Surg.* 1987;22(7):588–92.

Shimada K, Hosokawa S, Matsumoto F, Johnin K, Naitoh Y, Harada Y. Urological management of cloacal anomalies. *Int J Urol.* 2001;8(6):282–9.

Thomas DF. Cloacal malformations: embryology, anatomy and principles of management. *Prog Pediatr Surg.* 1989;23:135–43.

Warne S, Chitty LS, Wilcox DT. Prenatal diagnosis of cloacal anomalies. *BJU Int.* 2002; 89(1):78–81.

Warne SA, Wilcox DT, Creighton S, Ransley PG. Long-term gynecological outcome of patients with persistent cloaca. *J Urol.* 2003;170(4 pt 2):1493–6.

Warne SA, Wilcox DT, Ledermann SE, Ransley PG. Renal outcome in patients with cloaca. *J Urol.* 2002;167(6):2548–51; discussion 2551.

16 | Urinary Tract Infections

Kim A. R. Hutton

CASE 1

An 11-month-old girl was referred to the pediatric emergency assessment unit with a 10-day history of fever, vomiting, and more recent irritability. The general practitioner had previously made a clinical diagnosis of an upper respiratory viral illness and otitis media, which was treated with oral amoxicillin – a 7-day course had just been completed. On examination the infant was flushed, irritable, but easily placated with no rash or neck stiffness. Vital signs: temperature 38.8°C, pulse 170 beats/min, respiratory rate 40/min. Capillary return was less than 2 sec. The throat was mildly injected, the right ear drum was pink, and the left could not be seen due to wax. The chest was clear to auscultation, and abdominal examination was normal.

1 How would you investigate this infant?
2 Figure 16.1 illustrates five different ways of collecting a urine sample for culture. Which would be your first choice, and why?
3 Having made a diagnosis of urinary tract infection (UTI), what would be your preferred route and duration of antibiotic administration?
4 After successful treatment of the acute UTI, what advice would you give to the parents?
5 How would you attempt to prevent further UTI episodes, and what urological radiological investigations would you organize?

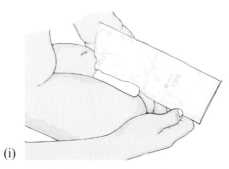

(i)

Fig. 16.1 Five different ways of collecting a urine sample.

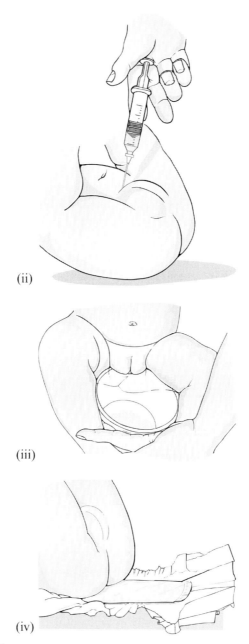

(ii)

(iii)

(iv)

Fig. 16.1 (*Contd.*)

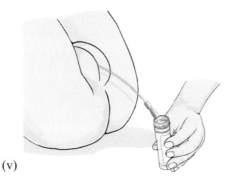

(v)

Fig. 16.1 (Contd.)

Discussion

1 As this child has no obvious cause for fever, an urgent urine sample must be collected and sent for culture. Clinicians assessing infants with pyrexia need to be aware that when a source for infection is not evident on history taking or clinical examination, a significant proportion (6.5% of girls and 3.3% of boys) will have an underlying UTI, and of these 10% will have a bacteraemia related to the same uropathogenic organism. Symptoms of UTI in young children are often nonspecific and include poor feeding, lethargy, irritability, fever, vomiting, weight loss, smelly urine, parental perception of dysuria, persistent jaundice in the neonate, failure to thrive, and fits. The key to diagnosis is to have a high index of suspicion and to investigate promptly. The clinical importance of UTI in small children is in their susceptibility to renal parenchymal damage and subsequent renal scarring, with a risk of future hypertension and, if severe and bilateral, of subsequent renal failure. Accurate and early detection with appropriate treatment and subsequent management should limit this morbidity.

2 There is controversy regarding the most appropriate method for urine collection in an infant suspected of having a UTI. The gold standard is suprapubic bladder aspiration, and samples via this route are not affected by urethral or periurethral (i.e. skin) contamination. Any number of gram negative bacilli and greater than a few thousand gram positive cocci per milliliter on culture signify a UTI. There are drawbacks, however, in that suprapubic aspiration is invasive and not always readily accepted by parents, nursing staff, or doctors and the fact that urine may not be successfully obtained (success rate 23–90%); the incidence of dry taps can be reduced by using ultrasound guidance (success rate 79–100%). Catheter specimens are useful for sick infants where antibiotics need to be started almost immediately and avoid some of the problems of suprapubic aspiration. Catheterization is performed after cleaning the genitalia and perineum with soap and water; the first few milliliters of urine drained is discarded before collecting the specimen to minimize contamination from urethral organisms. With colony counts less than 10^3/ml, infection is unlikely; with counts of 10^3–10^4/ml, samples should be repeated; and with counts greater than 10^4/ml, UTI is highly likely. However, catheterization can be traumatic and has the potential of introducing organisms into a previously sterile urinary tract. In a less ill infant where antibiotics are not required immediately, a clean-catch urine sample may be appropriate and has proven accuracy in detecting UTI in infancy. Colony-forming units of greater than 10^4/ml in a boy and greater than 10^5/ml in a girl make a UTI likely, although it is noted that definitions of positive and negative results are statistical and not absolute. Some samples may need repeating to obtain results related to the individual clinical situation. All of the above techniques are superior to pad or bag samples, which have a high contamination rate and should not be relied upon in making a diagnosis of UTI in acutely ill infants in the hospital setting.

3 Several studies have shown that oral antibiotics are safe and effective in the treatment of acute pyelonephritis in children over 1 month of age. Oral cefixime for 14 days (double dose on day 1) has been shown to be just as good in the treatment of children 1–24 months old with fever and UTI when compared with an initial 3-day intravenous cefotaxime followed by oral cefixime for 11 days. Amoxicillin-clavulanic acid given orally results in similar outcomes to intravenous therapy when comparing the time for defervescence, recurrence of UTI, or frequency of renal scintigraphy defects on follow-up. There is no evidence that extended intravenous therapy reduces subsequent renal scar development. In a child unable to take oral medication because of vomiting or in toxic infants with severe illness, intravenous fluids and antibiotics are obviously required. The choice of an antibiotic is dictated in part by knowledge of local bacterial resistance for community and hospital-acquired UTI. If gentamicin is one of the selected antimicrobials, current evidence supports once-daily dosing in pediatric practice, which simplifies administration and minimizes costs. A recent editorial suggests the following first-line oral antibiotics: trimethoprim alone or in combination with sulphamethoxazole, and cephalexin or amoxicillin-clavulanic acid. Obviously, antibiotic therapy is modified if required when bacterial sensitivities are available. The optimum duration of treatment is unknown, and further evidence-based data are required before traditional 7–14-day courses of antibiotics are discarded in favor of shorter duration of treatment (as often recommended in uncomplicated lower UTI in childhood).

Table 16.1 Uroprophylaxis for children with a diagnosis of UTI

Antimicrobial	Dose (mg/kg)	Frequency
Trimethoprim	1–2	At night
Nitrofurantoin	1–2	At night
Nalidixic acid	10	Twice a day
Cephalexin	10–15	At night

Infants under 1 month of age should have intravenous antibiotics because of the high incidence of associated bacteraemia and prevalence of underlying uropathy (obstructed systems, high-grade vesicoureteric reflux [VUR], duplex anomalies, posterior urethral valves). Intravenous cefotaxime or a beta lactam antibiotic and an aminoglycoside are indicated.

4 Parents need to be aware of a need for good fluid intake, be on the alert for further symptoms that might suggest a relapse or recurrence of UTI, and know what to do in such a situation. A repeat urine sample is required after completing the course of antibiotics to make sure that the infection has been cleared. Provision of written parent information leaflets on UTI is useful.

5 All infants with a diagnosed UTI should be started on prophylactic oral antibiotics once full dose treatment has finished and until investigations are completed (see Table 16.1). Guidelines for investigating children under 1 year in the United Kingdom are from the Royal College of Physicians Working Group 1991, who recommended an ultrasound of the kidneys and bladder, a plain abdominal radiograph to exclude renal stones and spinal defects, a micturating cystourethrogram (MCUG) when the urine was sterile, and a DMSA scan 3 months after the acute UTI episode. Most centers now omit the plain X-ray as stones are unlikely to be missed on modern ultrasound imaging and the spine can be assessed on postvoid MCUG frames. The American Academy of Pediatrics guidelines of 1999 recommend that infants and young children 2 months to 2 years of age should have a prompt ultrasound if response to treatment is inadequate after 48 hours. All other children should have an ultrasound at the earliest convenient time, and both groups are advised to undergo an MCUG or radionuclide cystography (not recommended for boys where urethral anatomy needs to be assessed, e.g. to exclude posterior urethral valves, or for girls with voiding dysfunction symptoms when not infected). Clinicians continue to question the appropriateness of these investigations; and in the light of increased prenatal detection of significant uropathies, some recent studies have argued that ultrasound in the first UTI may be unnecessary.

The girl in the case presented had a pad urine, which tested positive for nitrites and protein, and a clean-catch urine sample sent for culture. Microscopy showed 50–100 WBCs/cmm and bacteria. She was prescribed oral amoxicillin-clavulanic acid and was to be switched to oral trimethoprim when sensitivities revealed resistance with greater than 10^5 coliform organisms/ml and recovered well. A renal ultrasound was normal. MCUG revealed grade 2 right-sided VUR, and a DMSA 3 months later showed normal kidneys with no scarring. She was maintained on trimethoprim prophylaxis until out of nappies and has remained well and infection free.

Suggested reading

American Academy of Pediatrics. Practice parameter: the diagnosis, treatment, and evaluation of the initial urinary tract infection in febrile infants and young children. *Pediatrics.* 1999;103:843–52.

Bloomfield P, Hodson EM, Craig JC. Antibiotics for acute pyelonephritis in children. *Cochrane Database Syst Rev.* 2003;3:CD003772.

Craig JC, Hodson EM. Treatment of acute pyelonephritis in children. *BMJ.* 2004;328:179–80.

Hoberman A, Wald ER, Hickey RW, et al. Oral versus initial intravenous therapy for urinary tract infections in young febrile children. *Pediatrics.* 1999;104:79–86.

Zamir G, Sakran W, Horowitz Y, Koren A, Miron D. Urinary tract infection: is there a need for routine renal ultrasonography? *Arch Dis Child.* 2004;89:466–8.

CASE 2

An 11-year-old girl with a history of recurrent UTIs from the age of 3 was referred to the pediatric urology service. Investigation by the pediatrician at first presentation was with an ultrasound and DMSA scan. There was no evidence of upper tract dilatation, the right kidney was normal, and the left kidney was smaller with focal lower pole scarring. Differential function of the right kidney was 66%, and that of the left was 34%. A decision at that time was made to treat with prophylactic antibiotics and not proceed with an MCUG. Over the years she had continued to have recurrent UTIs, and the recent symptom complex was of pyrexia, left loin pain, and vomiting, with a couple of hospital admissions for intravenous antibiotics therapy.

1 How would you describe the type of infections this girl has?

2 What pathology is likely to be responsible for her continued problems?

3 What investigations have been performed, and what do they show (see Fig. 16.2)?

4 What measures might help reduce the chance of further UTI in this girl?

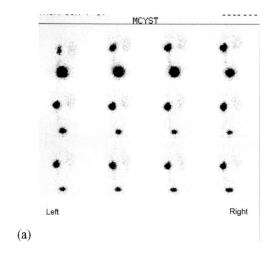

(a)

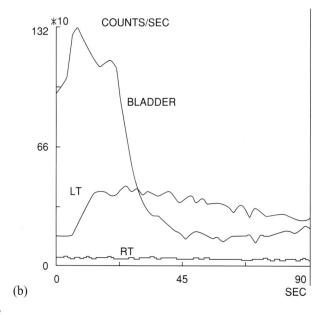

(b)

Fig. 16.2

Discussion

1 The history of pyrexia and vomiting suggests upper UTI as opposed to lower UTI, although distinguishing between the two on clinical grounds alone can be unreliable. Loin pain points to upper tract involvement, but an absence of loin pain or tenderness in a similar case would not exclude active pyelonephritis. Uncomplicated UTIs, in contrast, present as

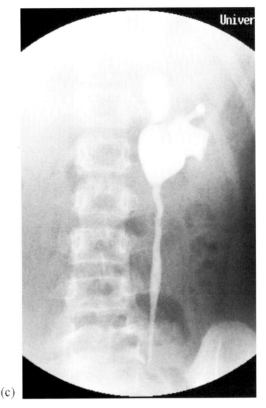

(c)

Fig. 16.2 (Contd.)

infective cystitis with lower tract symptoms of urinary frequency, urgency, dysuria, and foul-smelling urine. Antibiotic choice for acute episodes of infection in this girl should be guided by previous culture and sensitivity reports until up-to-date urine culture results are available. In the event of further infection, oral antibiotics continued for 7–10 days would be appropriate, assuming that clinical features suggest upper tract involvement. A short, 3–4 day course of antibiotics could be used for uncomplicated lower UTI.

2 She is likely to have underlying VUR. For decades, clinicians have recognized a relationship between UTI, VUR, and renal scarring, although a full understanding of the complex nature of these associations is still evolving. The incidence of childhood UTI is appreciable with 3.6% of boys and 11.3% of girls affected by their sixteenth birthday, with studies documenting renal scarring in up to 12% of cases. In addition, one-third of children investigated for a symptomatic UTI will have VUR, and a similar proportion of them will have parenchymal scarring on DMSA scanning. Not all children with scarred kidneys have VUR and host susceptibility, and bacterial virulence factors may be involved in some cases. Impaired bladder emptying may predispose to infection and be present in cases with dysfunctional voiding, neuropathic bladder, bladder outlet obstruction, VUR, or bladder diverticulum. Obstructive uropathies (e.g. PUJ obstruction, VUJ obstruction, duplex kidneys) predispose to UTI, as do urinary tract calculi. Recurrent infections may be related to underlying immunological problems or immunosuppression (kidney transplant recipients) or to an undiagnosed associated condition, e.g. diabetes mellitus. Bacterial factors may play a part, and so may adherence factors, and bacterial P fimbriae found on certain stains of *Escherichia coli* are known to be associated with acute pyelonephritis even in the absence of VUR.

3 Figure 16.2a shows posterior analog images, and Fig. 16.2b shows the time-activity curves for an indirect cystogram with reflux clearly visible on the left side extending to the renal pelvis. Figure 16.2c is a direct contrast MCUG, which revealed grade 2 left-sided reflux, with no detrusor abnormality, no bladder diverticulum, and normal bladder emptying. Although a direct contrast cystogram is more invasive and less well tolerated particularly at this age, it was requested to obtain anatomical detail prior to a planned interventional procedure.

4 Patients with VUR may have a reduced chance of further infection by increasing oral fluid intake, paying attention to a regular voiding pattern, and performing double or triple micturition. The later maneuver increases voiding efficiency by reducing residual urine volumes. Other medical measures used to reduce the incidence of recurrent UTI include prophylactic long-term antibiotics, oral cranberry products, and probiotics. A possible role for suitable vaccines in recurrent UTI is still to be fully explored. Although there are papers supporting regular low dose antibiotics in the prevention of recurrent UTI, a recent evidence-based review found that most studies had been poorly designed, with inherent biases likely to have overestimated the true treatment effect. It appears that large, randomized, double-blind, placebo-controlled trials are still required to determine whether antibiotic uroprophylaxis is indeed effective. There are two good-quality randomized controlled trials in women showing that cranberry products significantly reduce the incidence of UTIs, but whether these results are applicable to children is unclear. By definition, a probiotic is a "live microorganism which when administered in adequate amounts confers a health advantage to the host". The main species used is lactic acid bacteria, particularly *Lactobacillus* species, with the aim of restoring favorable commensal organisms in the gastrointestinal tract and perineum. UTI is

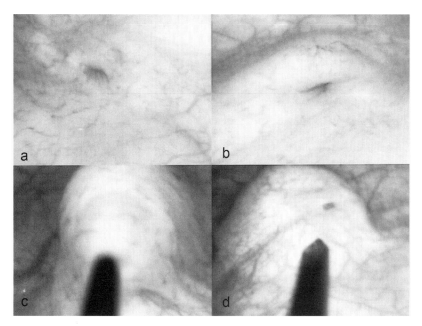

Fig. 16.3

usually an ascending infection caused by fecally derived bacteria, and 80% of the cases are related to *E. coli*. Rather disappointingly, interventional trials of probiotics have not been shown to prevent UTI, although it is possible that different products or different doses of the same products could be more successful.

The girl in the clinical case above underwent left-sided subureteric injection of Deflux performed cystoscopically under a general anesthetic (0.5ml injected, see Fig. 16.3). Follow-up ultrasound showed no hydronephrosis, and repeat MAG3 and indirect cystogram at 3 months and 1 year post treatment revealed no ongoing reflux. She has had no further episodes of UTI, is off all medications, and remains normotensive 4 years later at the age of 15. The literature relating to interventions for VUR is confusing, and debate continues on the most appropriate form of management: no treatment, long-term antibiotic prophylaxis, surgery, or a combination of antibiotic prophylaxis and surgery? In has been concluded in recent articles and evidence-based reviews that it is uncertain whether the identification of children with VUR is associated with clinically important benefit and that the additional benefit of surgery over antibiotics alone is at best small. However, in cases of breakthrough infection, surgery can on occasion provide very gratifying results.

Suggested reading

Fanos V, Cataldi L. Antibiotics or surgery for vesicoureteric reflux in children. *Lancet.* 2004;364:1720–2.

Jepson RG, Mihaljevic L, Craig J. Cranberries for preventing urinary tract infections. *Cochrane Database Syst Rev.* 2004;2:CD001321.

Kontiokari T, Nuutinen M, Uhari M. Dietary factors affecting susceptibility to urinary tract infection. *Pediatr Nephrol.* 2004;19:378–83.

Lambert H, Coulthard M. The child with urinary tract infection. In: Webb N, Postlethwaite R, eds. *Clinical Paediatric Nephrology.* 3rd ed. Oxford: Oxford University Press; 2003:197–226.

Williams GJ, Lee A, Craig JC. Long-term antibiotics for preventing recurrent urinary tract infection in children. *Cochrane Database Syst Rev.* 2001;4:CD001534.

CASE 3

A 9-year-old girl with a history of recurrent UTIs was referred to the outpatients. Her first UTI was at age 2, with several urinary infections since then. The symptoms were urinary frequency, smelly urine, and dysuria. The referring pediatrician had investigated with a renal ultrasound and DMSA scan, and these were normal. A MAG3 renogram and indirect cystogram showed no evidence of VUR.

1 What features of the history are going to be particularly important in assessing this girl's problem?
2 What aspects of the physical examination would you concentrate on?
3 On outpatient assessment the girl complains of current symptoms, suggesting a further UTI. Figure 16.4 shows two near-patient urine tests that have been performed. What are these, and how useful are these in diagnosing UTI?
4 How would you confirm the suspicion of a UTI?
5 How would you manage this patient?

Discussion

1 Information on fluid intake and voiding frequency are important, and obtaining a frequency/volume chart over a few days can be useful. Although bacteria probably ascend the urethra and gain access to the bladder in normal individuals, regular and complete bladder emptying prevents them from gaining a sufficient foothold to cause a UTI. Infrequent or incomplete emptying of the bladder is therefore likely to have an etiological role in some patients with recurrent infection. Other conditions linked to recurrent UTI include constipation, detrusor overactivity, and dysfunctional voiding. Asking questions regarding bowel habits, urinary frequency,

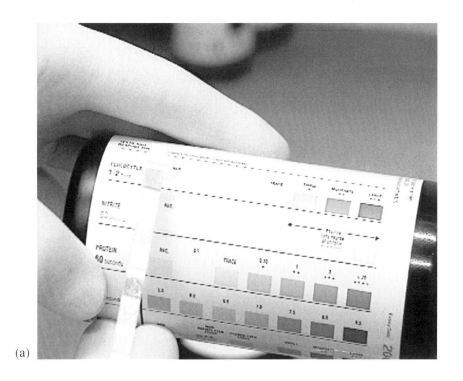

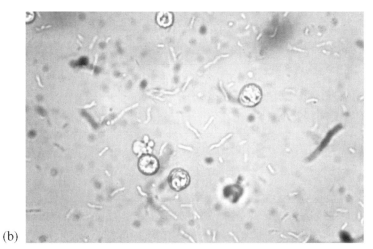

Fig. 16.4

urgency, urge incontinence, or diurnal incontinence may provide detail suggesting that these problems are involved in an individual patient's susceptibility to UTI. Are the stools passed small and hard? Is defecation painful? Are the bowels open less than once every 3 days? Does the child have to rush to the toilet or get caught short? Does she perform any unusual posturing (Vincent's curtsey sign) suggesting detrusor overactivity? Is there any associated wetting? Inadequate anogenital hygiene and toilet habits are thought to predispose to recurrent UTI. Are the underpants frequently contaminated with fecal material at the end of the day? Is the toilet paper passed back to front rather than front to back? Is the same piece of paper used more than once? Tight-fitting clothes and nylon underpants are thought to predispose to recurrent UTI. A recent study of 90 girls with recurrent UTI and a control group of 45 girls showed that infrequent voiding, poor fluid intake, and functional stool retention were significantly more frequent in girls with recurrent UTI, but inadequate stool hygiene or toilet habits were similar in both groups.

2 Abdominal examination may reveal a palpable bladder even if the patient has recently passed urine, suggestive of incomplete voiding. The colon may be loaded and indentable feces palpable in the rectum and sigmoid colon. Is there any perianal soiling or dampness in the underpants? If so, how long have the pants been on? The spine and genitalia should be examined, and a full neurological examination of the lower limbs should be performed to exclude possible neuropathy. What is the patient's gait like? Is there any evidence of pes cavus or clawing of the toes? Assess tone, power, coordination, sensation, position sense, reflexes, and plantar responses. However, in practice, it is rare to find any significant neurological abnormality.

3 Figure 16.4a shows reagent strip testing of urine. Various types are available, and the most useful for detecting UTI include a test for leucocyte esterase and nitrite. Leucocyte esterase is produced by white blood cells (WBCs) in the urine, and its presence raises the suspicion of a UTI. However, children can have a UTI without increased WBCs in the urine, and urinary WBCs can be increased without infection, e.g. with a fever from another source other than UTI. The test has a mean sensitivity of 83% and a mean specificity of 84%, and although it may be useful in suggesting UTI, there is a high false positive rate of up to 29%. The nitrite test detects the metabolism of nitrates to nitrites by bacteria in the urine and has a mean sensitivity of 50% and mean specificity of 98% (false positive rate of up to 5%). A positive nitrite stick test is, therefore, highly suggestive of infection, but a negative result in no way rules out a UTI – there is a high false negative rate. The reason for this is that some organisms do not convert urinary nitrate to nitrite, whereas others may take a few hours

to produce detectable levels of nitrite; with the frequency of micturition during a UTI, there may not be sufficient time for nitrite concentrations to rise sufficiently for a positive test result. If these two tests are combined and either is positive, the sensitivity increases to 88%. Figure 16.4b shows phase contrast microscopy of uncentrifuged fresh urine with bacterial rods visible together with white blood cells. A leucocyte concentration of greater than 10/cmm has a sensitivity for UTI of 77% and a false positive rate of 11%. The presence of organisms is highly suggestive of infection with a sensitivity of 93% and specificity of 95%.

4 A urine culture, usually a midstream specimen, is the only way to confirm a UTI. All near-patient tests have inherent false positive and false negative rates. Culture results are reported using Kass' original criteria of greater than 10^5 colony-forming units/ml as diagnostic of a UTI.

5 A urinary flow rate may give an indication of voiding dysfunction. For example, an interrupted flow pattern might suggest dysfunctional voiding, where there is external sphincter activity during a detrusor contraction, or represent abdominal straining due to detrusor failure – a feature of the "lazy bladder" syndrome. Renal and bladder ultrasound is useful for excluding any anatomical abnormality and measuring postvoid bladder residual volumes ($>10\%$ of expected bladder capacity is accepted as significant). Adequate fluid intake should be achieved and any constipation managed with oral stool softeners and laxatives such as lactulose, Senakot, or sodium picosulphate. Dietetic assessment and advice on dietary fiber intake may be appropriate. Symptoms of detrusor overactivity can be managed by avoiding caffeine intake and prescribing oral anticholinergics (oxybutynin or tolterodine). If bladder emptying is poor, double voiding, alpha-adrenergic blocking drugs (doxazocin), and, very occasionally, intermittent catheterization are required to reduce UTIs and control incontinence. Dysfunctional voiding may be helped by biofeedback techniques, and the management of these girls with recurrent UTIs and voiding problems is often facilitated by early involvement of a pediatric urology nurse specialist. Most patients will also be managed on low-dose prophylactic antibiotics to prevent further UTI. Medication is usually given at bedtime to provide adequate urinary drug concentrations during sleep when urine output is reduced and the patient is not routinely emptying the bladder. The drugs used are chosen for activity against urinary pathogens while having little effect on normal gut flora (sugar-free preparations are usually available). Routine advice often given by clinicians but not necessarily evidence based is for regular bathing, avoiding shampoo in the bath, bubble baths, and highly scented soaps and to dry carefully and use a barrier cream if there is local perineal/genital soreness.

The girl in the case above was noted to have a poor fluid intake and was an infrequent voider, going only 2–3 times per day. In addition, she had a postvoid residual of 44 ml. She was maintained on oral nitrofurantoin 1mg/kg at night and encouraged to perform regular timed voiding together with double micturition. Her infections stopped.

Suggested reading

Cain MP, Wu SD, Austin PF, Herndon CD, Rink RC. Alpha blocker therapy for children with dysfunctional voiding and urinary retention. *J Urol.* 2003;170:1514–15.

Gorelick MH, Shaw KN. Screening tests for urinary tract infection in children: A meta-analysis. *Pediatrics.* 1999;104:e54.

Loening-Baucke V. Urinary incontinence and urinary tract infection and their resolution with treatment of chronic constipation of childhood. *Pediatrics.* 1997;100:228–32.

Pohl HG, Bauer SB, Borer JG, et al. The outcome of voiding dysfunction managed with clean intermittent catheterization in neurologically and anatomically normal children. *BJU Int.* 2002;89:923–7.

Smellie JM, Katz G, Gruneberg RN. Controlled trial of prophylactic treatment in childhood urinary-tract infection. *Lancet.* 1978;2:175–8.

Stauffer CM, van der Weg B, Donadini R, Ramelli GP, Marchand S, Bianchetti MG. Family history and behavioral abnormalities in girls with recurrent urinary tract infections: a controlled study. *J Urol.* 2004;171:1663–5.

CASE 4

A girl with an antenatally detected uropathy was investigated postnatally with an ultrasound and MCUG, which showed bilateral hydroureteronephrosis and high-grade bilateral VUR (grade 5 on the left, grade 4 on the right). She was treated conservatively by the local pediatricians and commenced on prophylactic trimethoprim. She suffered a breakthrough UTI (infection while on oral uroprophylaxis) at 5 months of age and was treated at the local hospital with intravenous antibiotics; the cultured enterococcus organism was sensitive to trimethoprim, and so this was continued as the prophylactic agent. A further breakthrough UTI occurred at 9 months of age, again requiring parenteral antibiotics; this was resistant to trimethoprim and on the basis of sensitivities, prophylaxis was changed to nitrofurantoin. She had another breakthrough infection at 11 months of age requiring hospital admission and was referred to the pediatric nephrologists and surgeons.

1 Figure 16.5 shows a chart of this child's weight gain through the first year of life. What is going on?

2 What further investigations are required in this girl?

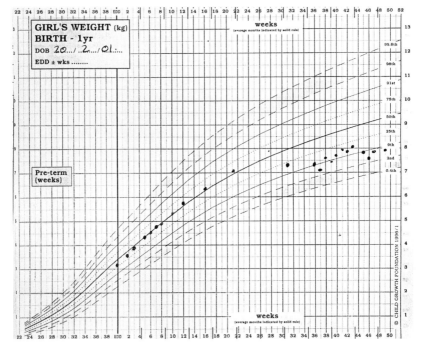

Fig. 16.5

3 What is the likely cause of her breakthrough infections?
4 How would you manage this patient?

Discussion

1 The growth chart shows normal progression along the 50th percentile for weight during the first 6 months of life. Thereafter her growth has faltered, with the plotted weight starting to cross centile lines; and at approximately 1 year of age the weight is noted to be below the 9th centile, confirming a clinical impression of failure to thrive. It is likely that the recurrent breakthrough infections are the underlying cause of this significant growth problem. Other causes, including a sweat test for cystic fibrosis, were investigated; all of these were normal.

2 Investigation should proceed as per published guidelines. The Royal College of Physicians recommend a DMSA in addition to an ultrasound and an MCUG in children under 1 year of age with a UTI. For children aged 1–6 years an ultrasound and a DMSA is advised (and a cystogram is confined to children with abnormalities on these investigations, history suggestive of pyelonephritis, family history of VUR, or recurrent infections),

199

whereas for children aged over 7 years with first UTI an ultrasound should be the only initial investigation required. Most physicians agree that all children should be investigated after a first UTI, but increasingly doctors are aware of the need to avoid unnecessary tests that are unlikely to alter management. Guidelines obviously require updating in the light of new evidence, and in the United Kingdom physicians are awaiting new NICE (the National Institute for Clinical Excellence) guidelines for the investigation and management of UTI in children; these guidelines are expected to be issued by November 2006. This girl's DMSA scan showed widespread scarring of both kidneys, with differential function of the right being 44% and that of the left being 56%.

3 The gross VUR is likely to be closely related to her susceptibility to recurrent UTI. Studies have shown a significant association between recurrent UTI, grade 3–5 VUR, and the presence of defects on DMSA scanning, with 60% of children in this group suffering breakthrough infection. Obviously if there is any possibility of underlying obstruction, a MAG 3 renogram should be performed, preferably with a urinary catheter in the bladder, as gross VUR can make interpretation of drainage curves difficult. There may be a problem with noncompliance in taking uroprophylaxis. In a situation of breakthrough infection with an organism sensitive to the prophylactic antibiotic, poor compliance is likely, and it is known that between one third and two thirds of patients have compliance problems. Urinary antimicrobial levels can be measured to document satisfactory compliance. Breakthrough UTI may be related to the development of bacterial resistance, in which case the UTI should be treated with an alternative suitable antibiotic; following successful treatment, prophylaxis should be switched with a new prophylactic agent to which the organism is sensitive. Host susceptibility factors may be present: it is known that blood group ABO, blood group p, Lewis antigen status, and secretor phenotype are related to UTI susceptibility, and some children have low urinary IgA levels. There is a familial susceptibility to UTI, and there is a 20–50-fold risk of VUR in children with a family history of VUR. The repeated use of antibiotics for other reasons (e.g. otitis media) may lead to alteration in bowel flora and recolonization with strains of bacteria that are more likely to cause symptomatic UTI.

4 She requires monitoring for the development of hypertension and proteinuria, together with assessment of overall renal function. A priority is to prevent further breakthrough UTI, because she is at risk of further renal scarring due to her young age (most acquired renal scarring occurs under the age of 4). A decision needs to be made as to whether the high-grade reflux should be corrected surgically. Assessment by the surgical team in this

case revealed a persistently distended bladder with poor emptying characteristics. Neurological examination and an MRI scan of the spine were normal. A ureteric reimplantation was not felt to be a suitable option at this stage because of her age and the significantly abnormal bladder emptying. An attempt to institute clean intermittent catheterization was not readily accepted, and therefore a decision was made to create a temporary vesicostomy. This was successful in preventing further UTI, stabilizing renal function and allowing her to thrive. She is now 3 year old, has learned urethral clean intermittent catheterization, and is awaiting urodynamic investigation prior to further surgery. If this patient had been a boy with primary VUR and recurrent breakthrough UTI, a circumcision could have been contemplated in an attempt to reduce further infection, as circumcised boys are known to have UTIs 10 times fewer than uncircumcised individuals.

Suggested reading

Royal College of Physicians Research Unit Working Group. Guidelines for the management of acute urinary tract infection in childhood. Report of Working Group of the Research Unit, Royal College of Physicians. *J R Coll Physicians Lond.* 1991;25:36-42.

Hutton KA, Thomas DF. Selective use of cutaneous vesicostomy in prenatally detected and clinically presenting uropathies. *Eur Urol.* 1998;33:405-11.

Mingin GC, Nguyen HT, Baskin LS. Abnormal dimercapto-succinic acid scans predict an increased risk of breakthrough infection in children with vesicoureteral reflux. *J Urol.* 2004;172:1075-7.

Panaretto K, Craig J, Knight J, Howman-Giles R, Sureshkumar P, Roy L. Risk factors for recurrent urinary tract infection in preschool children. *J Paediatr Child Health.* 1999;35:454-9.

Smyth AR, Judd BA. Compliance with antibiotic prophylaxis in urinary tract infection. *Arch Dis Child.* 1993;68:235-6.

CASE 5

KG was a very low birth weight premature neonate born at 26 weeks' gestation, was one of triplets, and weighed 740 g. In the first few weeks of life he suffered a number of the problems commonly encountered in infants of his size, including respiratory distress, recurrent sepsis treated with courses of intravenous antibiotics, possible necrotizing enterocolitis, and retinopathy of prematurity. At 3 weeks of age, during a further episode of presumed sepsis, he developed lower abdominal distension, stopped passing urine, and was thought to have a palpable bladder. An urgent renal tract ultrasound was performed.

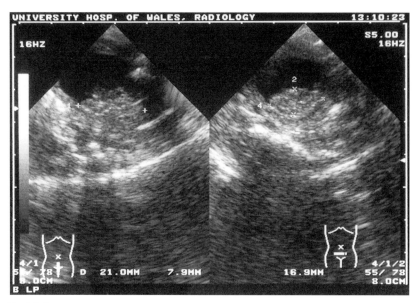

UNIVERSITY HOSP. OF WALES, RADIOLOGY   13:10:23

Fig. 16.6

1 What abnormality has been identified on this bladder scan (see Fig. 16.6)?
2 How would you confirm the diagnosis and manage the problem?
3 What other potential medical therapies are available?
4 If surgery is required, what procedure would you perform?

Discussion

1 There is an echogenic mass at the bladder base obstructing the internal urethral meatus, measuring $21 \times 8 \times 17$ mm, and consistent with a fungal ball. Other possible diagnoses include a bladder tumor or blood clot.

2 The bladder outflow obstruction needs to be relieved either by urethral or suprapubic catheterization. A urine sample is required for fungal culture and sensitivities. Routine bacterial culture should also be performed. Bloods tests for renal function and inflammatory markers should be obtained as a baseline and to follow subsequent response to treatment. Blood cultures should be taken to document any associated candidemia. This boy had a urethral catheter passed; urine microscopy showed budding yeasts and culture confirmed *Candida albicans* infection. Systemic antifungal treatment was started with amphotericin B (1 mg/kg/day) and fluconazole (6 mg/kg/day). Fungi are normal saphrophytic flora in healthy individuals, and when infection occurs in a neonate it usually manifests itself as an innocent nappy rash or an episode of oral thrush. On occasion, however, severe systemic disease can develop with *C. albicans* and *C. parapsilosis* as the predominant pathogenic species. Renal tract candidiasis is a rare but well-recognized complication of neonatal intensive care, and systemic fungal infection in neonates is life threatening, with mortality rates of 34–70%. Risk factors for infection include prematurity, malnutrition, prior antibiotic exposure, endotracheal intubation, presence of a central venous or umbilical artery catheter, total parenteral nutrition, and underlying immunosuppression. Primary sites of the disease include the bloodstream, urinary tract, meninges, lungs, and bone, although disseminated infection with multiorgan involvement is common. The incidence of systemic candidiasis in neonates weighing 1500 g or less is 4%, with approximately 10% of infants less than 1000 g being affected. Candida UTI can be an ascending infection in association with underlying structural or drainage problems, or it can result from the presence of an indwelling catheter. More usually, renal tract involvement is secondary to generalized systemic disease and hematogenous spread; patients with unobstructed systems respond to systemic antifungal therapy. Complications include renal and perirenal abscess formation and obstruction due to fungal bezoars. The clinician must suspect fungal balls in all neonates with systemic candidiasis or candiduria and in patients at high risk of fungal infection when unexplained oliguria, anuria, hypertension, or a renal mass develops. Diagnosis is with ultrasound, which may reveal hydronephrosis, increased cortical echogenicity, and echogenic nonshadowing material in the collecting system. Obstructing candidiasis usually affects the kidneys (PUJ obstruction) which if bilateral results in anuria and acute renal failure. Obstructed systems require percutaneous nephrostomy drainage, and percutaneous nephroscopic removal of obstructing fungal balls has been described in the literature. Occasionally, open pyelotomy with removal of fungal balls or fungal casts of the collecting system, open nephrostomy placement, or even nephrectomy is required to control infection. Severe retroperitoneal and ureteral disease can result in ureteral loss and a need for subsequent reconstructive surgery. Systemic antifungal treatment should continue until two clear urine cultures are obtained 1 week apart. It has been noted that radiological evidence of fungal balls can persist long after the urine has been rendered sterile and should not dictate the duration of antifungal therapy. Liposomal amphotericin B has been shown to be an effective and safe treatment of candidemia in premature infants and probably has fewer side effects compared with standard amphotericin B (less nephrotoxicity). Itraconazole has been compared with fluconazole in a randomized double-blind trial and found to be as effective in treating nosocomial candidiasis in children receiving pediatric intensive care. Amphotericin can only be given intravenously, whereas fluconazole can be administered orally or intravenously, with approximately 80% of the drug excreted remaining unchanged as active drug in the urine.

3 Mechanical disruption of bladder fungal balls has been reported using amphotericin B bladder irrigation. This was attempted in our case with no effect, and repeated bladder irrigation with an amphotericin B solution (5 mg/100 ml) also failed to dissolve the fungal bezoars. Bladder installations of a streptokinase solution (15,000 IU in 5 ml instilled twice a day via the urinary catheter with catheter clamping for 1 hour, then free drainage repeated for 3 days) was also unsuccessful. There are, however, a number of reports documenting successful management of upper tract fungal balls with nephrostomy irrigation (either intermittent or continuous, one or two nephrostomies with in and out irrigation) using amphotericin (the concentration of amphotericin solution used, frequency, and duration of therapy not standardized) and two publications describing successful streptokinase use in treating therapy-resistant renal fungal balls.

4 Surgical removal of the obstructing fungal mass was indicated because of bezoar persistence and continued bladder outflow obstruction. Possible therapeutic approaches included cystourethroscopy and transurethral removal, suprapubic percutaneous retrieval using direct transurethral visualization (both techniques precluded because of the size of our patient

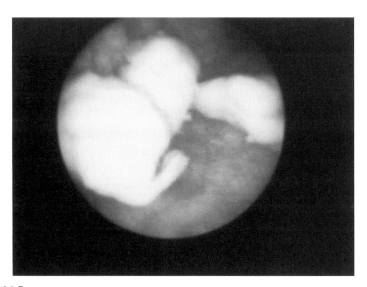

Fig. 16.7

and lack of suitable miniature cystourethroscopes), percutaneous bladder access, and suprapubic endoscopic removal or vacuum extraction or open surgical removal. Because of the infant's very small size, blind insertion of a suprapubic port into the bladder was felt to be unsafe. A small cystotomy to obtain safe access to the bladder interior was performed under general anesthesia, an excellent view of the fungal balls was achieved using an 8.5FG cystoscope (see Fig. 16.7), and successful retrieval of the putty-like fungal masses was achieved endoscopically using 3FG alligator forceps. Follow-up ultrasounds showed no residual bezoars, and Candida infection was cleared with systemic antifungal agents. KG is now 2 years and 10 months old and has an essentially normal renal tract.

Suggested reading

Babu R, Hutton KA. Renal fungal balls and pelvi-ureteric junction obstruction in a very low birth weight infant: treatment with streptokinase. *Pediatr Surg Int*. 2004;20:804–5.

Baetz-Greenwalt B, Debaz B, Kumar ML. Bladder fungus ball: a reversible cause of neonatal obstructive uropathy. *Pediatrics*. 1988;81:826–9.

Benjamin DK Jr, Fisher RG, McKinney RE Jr, Benjamin DK. Candidal mycetoma in the neonatal kidney. *Pediatrics*. 1999;104:1126–9.

Chapman RL. Candida infections in the neonate. *Curr Opin Pediatr*. 2003;15:97–102.

Redman JF, Lightfoot ML, Reddy PP. Extensive upper and mid ureteral loss in newborns: experience with reconstruction in 2 patients. *J Urol*. 2002;168:691–3.

17 | Ambiguous Genitalia and Intersex Conditions

Prasad Godbole and Peter Cuckow

Introduction

Sexual determination is a complex process that occurs in an organized sequential manner. When chromosomal, gonadal, or phenotypic sex determination goes awry, intersexuality develops. Classification of such abnormalities is usually arbitrary but may be based on abnormalities of gonadal determination (usually due to sex chromosomal defects) and abnormalities of genital differentiation such as masculinization of a genetic female or undervirilization of a genetic male (female and male pseudohermaphrodites, respectively). The management of intersex conditions needs a multidisciplinary approach between pediatric endocrinologists, pediatric urologists, geneticists, psychologists, and a dedicated team of nurse specialists. As controversy rages in the role of surgery for certain conditions such as congenital adrenal hyperplasia (CAH) or determination of sex of rearing in cloacal exstrophy, it is imperative that the parents be actively involved in the decision-making process. The following problems give an overview of some of the intersex conditions that may be encountered in clinical practice.

CASE 1

A newborn is referred to you with ambiguous genitalia. On examination, he has a severe penoscrotal hypospadias, marked chordee (Fig. 17.1), and palpable undescended gonads. The karyotype is 46,XY.

1 Describe the normal sex development.
2 What is the differential diagnosis in this case?
3 How would you investigate this newborn?
4 He is noted to have a large prostatic utricle, which is discovered when he has a cystoscopy. When would you operate on this? What are the various surgical approaches?

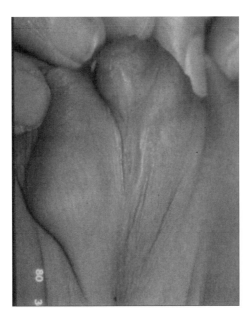

Fig. 17.1

Discussion

1 Normal sex development consists of three sequential processes, namely determination of genetic sex, determination of gonadal sex, and finally differentiation into the phenotypic sex (Fig. 17.2). The genetic sex is determined at the time of fertilization by the sex chromosome constitution. This genetic information determines differentiation into either a testis or ovary. Phenotypic sex is a result of male differentiation resulting from testicular hormone production: the anti-Müllerian hormone (AMH) produced by the Sertoli cells inhibits the Müllerian ducts, and testosterone produced by the Leydig cells stabilizes the Wolffian ducts. Testosterone is transformed into dihydrotestosterone, which is responsible for virilization of the external genitalia. Almost all of the steps of sex differentiation are under genetic control; mutation in any one may hence result in intersex abnormalities.

2 This case illustrates an example of a male pseudohermaphrodite (MPH) with incomplete masculinization. Although the differential diagnosis is long, it can be divided into impaired gonadotrophic action or function, impaired androgen biosynthesis, metabolism or action, impaired testosterone metabolism, androgen receptor defects, impaired AMH production, and syndromic associations of MPH. A detailed list is of abnormalities in

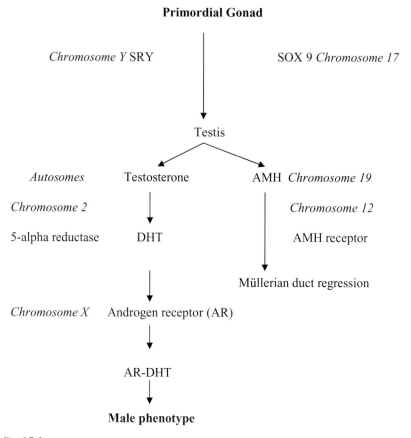

Primordial Gonad

Chromosome Y SRY   SOX 9 *Chromosome 17*

Testis

Autosomes   Testosterone   AMH *Chromosome 19*

Chromosome 2   *Chromosome 12*

5-alpha reductase   DHT   AMH receptor

Müllerian duct regression

Chromosome X   Androgen receptor (AR)

AR-DHT

Male phenotype

Fig. 17.2

male androgenization is given below. Not all abnormalities relate specifi-
cally to this case.

  a. Impaired gonadotrophic action or function: Leydig cell hypoplasia or
aplasia

  b. Impaired androgen biosynthesis

     Impaired testosterone biosynthesis

     Deficient formation of pregnenolone

     3-beta hydroxysteroid dehydrogenase deficiency

     17-alpha hydroxylase deficiency

     17-beta hydroxysteroid dehydrogenase deficiency

     Impaired testosterone metabolism

     5-alpha reductase deficiency

     Androgen receptor defects

     Partial or complete androgen insensitivity syndromes

   c. Impaired AMH production
        Persistent Müllerian duct syndromes
   d. Syndromic associations
        Absence of ductus deferens, epididymis, seminal vesicle, kidney, and
          ureter on one side
        Aniridia-Wilms tumor association
        Cloacal exstrophy
        Fraser's syndrome
3 The initial step would be to confirm an MPH by determining the karyotype (in this case 46,XY). Either an ultrasound or laparoscopy and cystoscopy or both should exclude Müllerian duct derivatives. Presence of
  Müllerian duct structures suggests a peristent Müllerian duct syndrome.
  This may be found in association with anomalies of testicular differentiation in conditions such as Denys-Drash syndrome, WAGR syndrome, XY
  gonadal dysgenesis, mixed gonadal dysgenesis, and testicular regression
  syndromes.
     Absence of Müllerian structures suggests an abnormality of androgen
  biosynthesis, metabolism, or action. Investigations are therefore tailored
  to these etiologies. They would include a human chorionic gonadotropin
  (HCG) stimulation test, testosterone basal and response as well as precur-
  sors, ACTH test, studies to detect genetic mutations along the biosynthetic
  and metabolic pathway, and receptor studies. The pediatric endocrinolo-
  gist would usually oversee these investigations.
4 Presence of a prostatic utricle in itself is not an indication for surgery. A
  utriculus may act as a reservoir leading to recurrent urinary tract infections or voiding disturbances. In these circumstances, excision is recommended. This can be performed laparoscopically or via the transvesical
  transtrigonal route.

Suggested reading

Forest MG. Ambiguous genitalia/intersex: endocrine aspects. In: Gearhart JP, Rink RR,
  Mouriquand P, eds. *Pediatric Urology*. Philadelphia: Saunders; 2001:623–58.
Hyun G, Kolon TF. A practical approach to intersex in the newborn period. *Urol Clin North
  Am*. 2004;31(3):435–43.
Morel Y, Rey R, Teinturier C, et al. Aetiological diagnosis of male sex ambiguity: a collab-
  orative study. *Eur J Pediatr*. 2002:161(1):49–59.
Willetts IE, Roberts JP, MacKinnon AE. Laparoscopic excision of a prostatic utricle in a
  child. *Pediatr Surg Int*. 2003;19(7):557–8.
Hadziselimovic F, Huff D. Gonadal differentiation – normal and abnormal testicular devel-
  opment. *Adv Exp Med Biol*. 2002;511:15–21.

CASE 2

A newborn baby is transferred to your department with ambiguous genitalia (Fig. 17.3). No gonads are palpable.

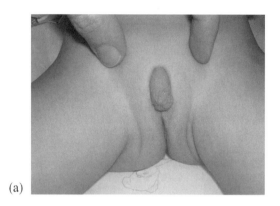

(a)

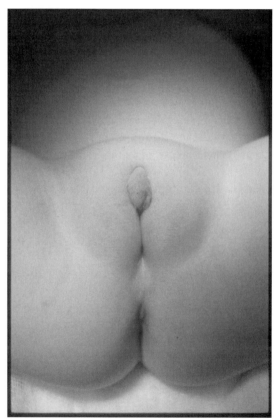

(b)

Fig. 17.3

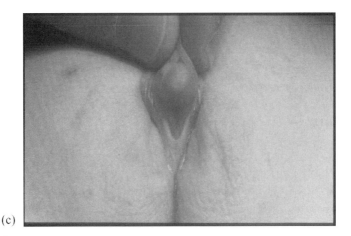

(c)

Fig. 17.3

1 Describe the features seen and the differential diagnosis.
2 What are the immediate concerns in the first few days of life?
3 What initial investigations are necessary? What subsequent investigations may you perform?
4 What are the controversies regarding feminizing genitoplasty in CAH?

Discussion

1 The features demonstrate a hypertrophied phallus, scrotalization (pigmentation and fusion) of the labial folds, and a common urogenital sinus (UGS). The differential diagnosis is that of an overvirilized female (female pseudohermaphrodite). The commonest cause of female pseudohermaphroditism (FPH) is inborn errors of biosynthesis in the cortisol and aldosterone pathway. Congenital adrenal adrenal hyperplasia accounts for up to 90% of cases. Other causes include maternal exposure to androgens during pregnancy and FPH associated with other malformations.

A list of the causes of overvirilization in an XX female is given below.

a. Inborn errors of cortisol metabolism
 Congenital adrenal hyperplasia
 21-hydroxylase deficiency
 11-beta hydroxylase deficiency
 3-beta hydroxysteroid dehydrogenase deficiency
b. Maternal exposure to androgens
 Adrenal or ovarian tumors
 Maternal ingestions of androgens or progestagens
c. FPH associated with other malformations

2 CAH due to 21-hydroxylase deficiency is the commonest cause of FPH. It may occur in its classic form or nonclassic form. In its classic form, it may present with deficient aldosterone synthesis and therefore a salt-wasting crisis. Hence early and close monitoring of serum biochemistry is essential. If the aldosterone synthesis is normal, it may present as a simple virilizing form. In the nonclassic form, signs of virilization are usually absent at birth and are usually evident in later childhood.

3 CAH occurs as a result of enzymatic deficiency in three basic steps in cortisol metabolism. The absence of palpable gonads, the presence of Müllerian structures, and an elevated 17-hydroxyprogesterone level in an XX female suggest the diagnosis of CAH due to 21-hydroxylase deficiency or 11-beta hydroxysteroid deficiency. A normal 17-OH progesterone level in this case would suggest CAH due to aromatase deficiency. Normal 17-OH progesterone levels but an abnormal karyotype (XO/XY, XX/XY, and XY) would suggest MPH with gonadal dysgenesis or true hermaphroditism. Hence in the first instance, careful clinical examination, ultrasound of the pelvis, 17-OH progesterone assay, and a karyotype are sufficient to make a diagnosis.

Subsequent investigations are aimed toward surgery. Anatomical knowledge of the UGS and the length of the common channel is essential and may be obtained by a careful cystovaginoscopy with or without a genitogram.

4 Surgery for CAH is currently under intense debate. The debate revolves around the need for surgery (both clitoral surgery and vaginoplasty), the long-term psychosocial and sexual outcome, the influence of intersex support groups, the parents' perspective, and more importantly the child's right to make a decision.

Clitoral surgery has moved from clitoral resection (no longer acceptable), clitoral recession (troublesome painful erections) to clitoral reduction. Preservation of the neurovascular bundle may preserve sensation according to some reports. However, more recently, studies suggest that a significant number of women who have had clitoral surgery as a baby suffer problems with altered sensation, sexual dissatisfaction, and anorgasmia. The authors preserve the urethral plate at the time of clitoral reduction to preserve circumferential innervation; however, long-term results will be many years to come. A significantly hypertrophied clitoris can cause disturbances in parental bonding with the child and social integration within the family. Hence in these cases, after a full discussion with the parents, clitoral surgery may be undertaken.

A vaginoplasty is performed to ensure that penetration and sexual intercourse may occur. There are two widely held views regarding the timing of vaginoplasty. Proponents of early vaginoplasty believe that concomitant clitoral and vaginal surgery is acceptable with good cosmetic results. Opponents to this view cite the high incidence of reoperations, especially at the time of puberty after neonatal or infant vaginoplasty, and therefore recommend a wait-and-watch policy till the child is Gillick competent to make her own decision.

There is no consensus view regarding feminizing genitoplasty surgery for CAH. Any decision regarding surgery should be in a multidisciplinary setting with full and active involvement of the parents in the decision-making process.

Suggested reading

Creighton SM, Minto CL, Liao LM, Alderson J, Simmonds M.
Meeting between experts: evaluation of the first UK forum for lay and professional experts in intersex. *Patient Educ Couns.* 2004;54(2):153–7.
Minto CL, Liao LM, Woodhouse CR, Ransley PG, Creighton SM. The effect of clitoral surgery on sexual outcome in individuals who have intersex conditions with ambiguous genitalia: a cross-sectional study. *Lancet.* 2003;361(9365):1252–7.
Rangecroft L, on behalf of the British Association of Paediatric Surgeons Working Party on the Surgical Management of Children Born With Ambiguous Genitalia. Surgical management of ambiguous genitalia. *Arch Dis Child.* 2003;88(9):799–801.
Schober JM, Meyer-Bahlburg HF, Ransley PG. Self-assessment of genital anatomy, sexual sensitivity and function in women: implications for genitoplasty. *BJU Int.* 2004;94(4):589–94.
Stikkelbroeck NM, Beerendonk CC, Willemsen WN, et al. The long term outcome of feminizing genital surgery for congenital adrenal hyperplasia: anatomical, functional and cosmetic outcomes, psychosexual development, and satisfaction in adult female patients. *J Pediatr Adolesc Gynecol.* 2003;16(5):289–96.

CASE 3

A 3-month-old girl presents with an irreducible left inguinal hernia (Fig. 17.4). At surgical exploration, she is noted to have presence of a testis in the hernial sac.
1 What are your surgical options?
2 What further investigations are necessary, and why?
3 What further surgical procedures may be necessary?

Discussion

1 The most important part of the surgery is the management of the irreducible hernia. This case illustrates a phenotypic female with

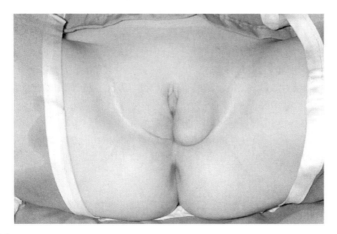

Fig. 17.4

intra-abdominal testis. This girl is going to require investigations as for a male pseudohermaphrodite. The testicle may be resected for histology (to detect presence of ovarian tissue) or may be returned back to the abdominal cavity pending further investigations and a plan of management. In either case the parents should be informed in detail about the findings and the need for further investigations.

2 The most likely diagnosis in this case is that of a complete androgen insensitivity syndrome (CAIS). CAIS may present in infants with an inguinal hernia and a palpable gonad, which turns out to be the testis. Müllerian structures are absent, and the vagina is short and blind ending. Investigations required for the diagnosis are a karyotype (XY), ultrasound of the pelvis, testosterone levels (usually high at puberty and in neonates), and androgen receptor and postreceptor studies on cultured genital skin fibroblasts (these may be receptor negative or receptor positive but qualitatively abnormal receptors). Following biochemical investigations, laparoscopy may be considered to exclude Müllerian structures and if orchiectomy is contemplated.

3 Gender assignment is confirmed as female in CAIS, and hence the need to perform bilateral orchidectomy due to the potential for development of gonadal tumors. This may be done via either the open or laparoscopic routes. The timing of surgery is controversial; however, some authorities feel that early orchiectomy may confer some positive psychological advantages versus a delayed decision for surgery. Estrogen replacement therapy is required at puberty. The short vagina may be suitable in most instances for dilatation, thus avoiding the need for reconstructive vaginal surgery.

Suggested reading

Barthold JS, Kumasi-Rivers K, Upadhyay J, Shekarriz B, Imperato-Mcginley J. Testicular position in the androgen insensitivity syndrome: implications for the role of androgens in testicular descent. *J Urol.* 2000;164(2):497–501.

Brinkmann A, Jenster G, Ris-Stalpers C. Molecular basis of androgen insensitivity. *Steroids.* 1996;61:172–75.

Minto CL, Liao KL, Conway GS, Creighton SM. Sexual function in women with complete androgen insensitivity syndrome. *Fertil Steril.* 2003;80(1):157–64.

Wilson JD. Syndromes of androgen resistance. *Biol Reprod.* 1992;46:168–73.

CASE 4

A newborn baby is transferred to your department with the following condition (Fig. 17.5).

1 What is the diagnosis?

2 How can this condition be diagnosed antenatally?

3 What are the current views regarding gender assignment in this condition?

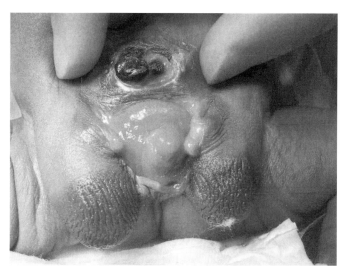

Fig. 17.5

Discussion

1 This baby has cloacal exstrophy, the severest form of the exstrophy-epispadias sequence. Typically, as in this case, the elephant trunk appearance can be seen, with the central exstrophied cecum and terminal ileum flanked on either side by a hemibladder. An omphalocele can be seen on the superior aspect. The phallus is bipartite.

2 Antenatally the absence of visualization of a bladder, a large infraumbilical midline anterior wall defect or cystic anterior wall structure, and an omphalocele with or without a myelomeningocele are seen in the majority of cases. Associated features may include lower extremity defects, renal anomalies, ascitis, hydrocephalus, or a narrow thorax.

3 Gender assignment or reassignment has remained the most controversial issue in the management of babies with cloacal exstrophy and remains the ultimate challenge. Traditionally, for the last 25 years, XY boys with cloacal exstrophy were gender reassigned in the neonatal period if the bipartite phallus was deemed to be too small to be functionally adequate after reconstruction. Boys underwent closure of the cloacal exstrophy and bilateral orchidectomy and future surgical reconstruction in keeping with a female gender. However, biological factors in the prenatal period may play a significant role in gender identification, especially due to brain imprinting with testosterone. The decision to assign a sex is guided by the prognosis of the "optimal" sex for the newborn, of which the elements are an overall sex-appropriate appearance with a stable gender identity; good sexual function, preferably combined with reproductive function if attainable; minimal medical procedures; and a reasonably happy life, given the limitations.

Recent longitudinal studies of males with severe phallic inadequacy who are gender reassigned or those with cloacal exstrophy have shown that a high proportion of these "females" gender reassigned back to males later in life and considered themselves male with male attitudes. Those who remained female had interests and attitudes that were more male in nature.

The issue of gender reassignment therefore remains a very delicate and sensitive issue. There is no clear-cut answer and any decision made must be in full consultation with the parents, pediatric endocrinologists, pediatric psychologist or psychiatrist, and pediatric urologists who are part of a dedicated team to manage such conditions. Newer techniques and advances in penile reconstruction in childhood and later life may play a role in the decision-making process.

Suggested reading

Diamond M, Sigmundson HK. Sex reassignment at birth. Long term review and clinical implications. *Arch Pediatr Adolsc Med.* 1997;151:298–304.
Nelson CP, Gearhart JP. Current views on evaluation, management, and gender assignment of the intersex infant. *Nat Clin Pract Urol.* 2004;1(1):38–43.

Reiner WG. Psychosexual development in genetic males assigned female: the cloacal exstrophy experience. *Child Adolesc Psychiatr Clin N Am.* 2004;13(3):657–74.

Reiner WG, Gearhart JP. Discordant sexual identity in some genetic males with cloacal exstrophy assigned to female sex at birth. *N Engl J Med.* Jan 2004;350(4):333–41.

Reiner WG, Kropp BP. A 7-year experience of genetic males with severe phallic inadequacy assigned female. *J Urol.* 2004;172(6 pt 1):2395–8.

Schober JM, Carmichael PA, Hines M, Ransley PG. The ultimate challenge of cloacal exstrophy. J Urol. 2002;167(1):300–4.

CASE 5

A 3-month-old boy is referred to you as his parents are concerned about his penile length, which they feel is too short. He has been seen by his family physician, who feels he may have a micropenis.

1 What is the differential diagnosis, and how can a micropenis be suspected on clinical grounds?

2 If a micropenis is suspected, what investigations might be performed and why?

3 What is the role of exogenous testosterone in micropenis?

4 What is the long-term outlook for males with micropenis or those that have been gender reassigned?

Discussion

1 A *micropenis* is defined as one where the stretched penile length (SPL) is 2 standard deviations below the reference range for age. It has to be differentiated from a buried penis, where the penis appears small due to the generous amount of fat and inner preputial skin that "buries" it (Fig. 17.6). The other condition that may be mistaken for a micropenis is a webbed penis, where there is encroachment of the scrotum onto the ventral aspect of the penile shaft. To determine the stretched penile length, the glans is grasped firmly and the length is measured from the tip of the glans to the pubic symphysis with a rigid ruler. The foreskin should not be measured. At birth an SPL of 1.9 cm or less is suggestive of a micropenis and needs investigation.

2 Development of the male genitalia is completed by 14 weeks of gestation. Initial testosterone secretion for the first 3 months is via the influence of placental HCG. From the fourth month, testosterone is secreted by the testis under the influence of gonadotropin-releasing hormones (GnRH) from the hypothalamus via the pituitary (follicle-stimulating hormone [FSH] and luteinizing hormone [LH]). Testosterone is converted to

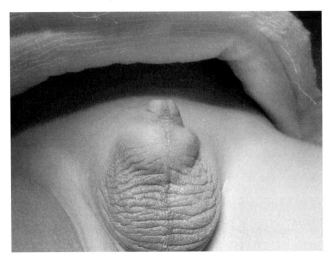

Fig. 17.6

5-dihydrotestosterone (DHT) by 5-alpha reductase. 5-DHT is responsible for the development of male external genitalia. A micropenis may result from the following:

a. Inadequate secretion of GnRH (hypogonadotrophic hypogonadism)

    Kallmann's syndrome (genitoolfactory dysplasia)

    Prader-Willi syndrome

    Laurence Moon Biedl syndrome.

b. Primary testicular failure (hypergonadotrophic hypogonadism)

    Gonadal dysgenesis

    Rudimentary testis syndrome

    Vanishing testis syndrome

c. LH receptor defects

d. Idiopathic micropenis

The aim of initial investigation is to differentiate between the two main causes of micropenis. A careful clinical examination including SPL, scrotum, and testes, as well as hypotonia (Prader-Willi syndrome), is performed. A karyotype should be performed to exclude major chromosomal abnormalities such as Klinefelter's syndrome. Depending on age, a cranial ultrasound or magnetic resonance imaging will give the anatomy of the hypothalamus and pituitary. Pituitary endocrine testing in the form of blood sugar, growth hormone (GH), serum electrolytes, and TFT, should be performed and early hormone replacement therapy commenced as necessary.

If testicular failure is the presumed diagnosis, endocrine testicular function should be assessed. This should include baseline testosterone and LH and FSH levels after HCG stimulation. Persistence of baseline testosterone levels but rises in FSH and LH levels after HCG stimulation suggest testicular failure. Recently assays of AMH (Müllerian inhibiting substance) have been described as being specific for functioning testicular tissue. If the testes are impalpable, a laparoscopy should be performed. If there is evidence of increase in testosterone levels after HCG stimulation and impalpable testis, a laparoscopy and the single or first stage of a Fowler Stephens orchidopexy should be performed.

3 Following diagnosis and initial management, the response of the penis to exogenous testosterone is determined. This may be evident at the time of the initial HCG stimulation test. In testicular failure, intramuscular testosterone may be used to demonstrate response. In hypogonadotrophic hypogonadism, there was controversy with respect to early use of testosterone as this was demonstrated to prevent further response to testosterone at puberty in mice. However, recently, long-term studies of men with micropenis have found that use of testosterone during puberty and early adulthood help the penis achieve an SPL within 2 standard deviations of what is normal for age.

4 In cases of micropenis unresponsive to early testosterone therapy, gender reassignement was occasionally performed necessitating extensive surgical reconstruction. One long-term outcome study did not demonstrate any correlation between the SPL of micropenis in infancy and adulthood. All men in this study had a mean SPL within 2SD for their age. This could have been due to a greater than average interval SPL growth or the use of androgens. Another study of 20 males with micropenis unresponsive to androgens followed up into adulthood showed a persistent micropenis in 90% of them. All had a male gender identity; however 25% were undergoing psychiatric counseling due to fear of sexual rejection. Eight had not pursued any sexual activity. In another study of 13 males and 5 women (gender reassigned), 50% of men and 80% of women were dissatisfied with their genitalia. All men and 3 women were sexually active. All men and women had appropriate gender role identity.

Hence gender reassignment is not routinely recommended in boys with micropenis, because, although the results may be satisfactory, this requires extensive feminizing surgery. Controversy also exists in the role of fetal brain imprinting with testosterone and hence its implication on gender identity in those reared as females. Phallic lengthening reconstructive procedures if necessary may play a role in the future.

Suggested reading

Bin-Abbas B, Conte FA, Grumbach MM, Kaplan SL. Congenital hypogonadotrophic hypogonadism and micropenis: effect of testosterone treatment on adult penile size. Why sex reversal is not indicated. *J Pediatr*. 1999;134(5):579–83.

Husmann DA. The androgen insensitive micropenis: long-term follow-up into adulthood. *J Pediatr Endocrinol Metab*. 2004;17(8):1037–41.

Lee PA, Houk CP. Outcome studies among men with micropenis. *J Pediatr Endocrinol Metab*. 2004;17(8):1043–53.

Williams-Ashman HG, Reddi AH. Differentiation of mesenchymal tissues during phallic morphogenesis with emphasis on the penis: role of androgens and other regulatory agents. *J Steroid Biochem Mol Biol*. 1991;39:873–81.

Wisniewski AB, Migeon CJ, Gearhart JP, et al. Congenital micropenis: long-term medical, surgical and psychosexual follow-up of individuals raised male or female. *Horm Res*. 2001;56(1–2):3–11.

Index

Page numbers in *italic* represent figures, those in **bold** represent tables.

221